THE

AilamA®

EMOTIONAL

COOKBOOK AND NUTRITION PROGRAM

89 Quick and Easy Recipes for Sincere Eating

All Year Around

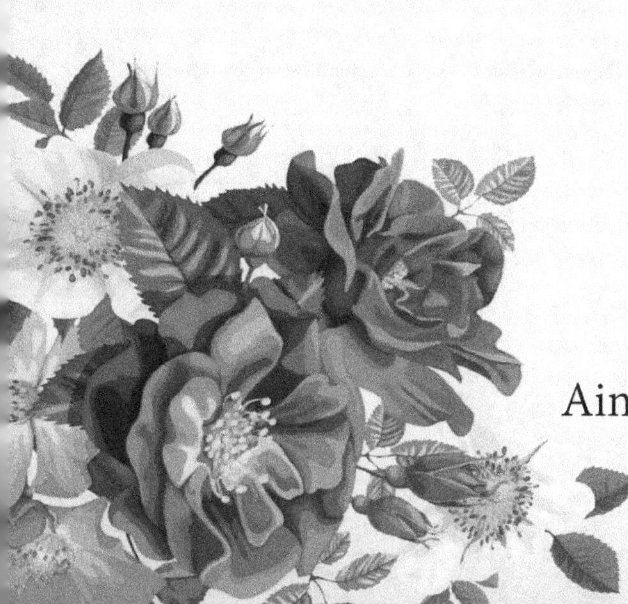

Aimee T. L. Kathartt

CONTENTS

Introduction 1
About The AilamA® Cookbook 3
A. The AilamA® Cookbook Recommends 3
  1. Meat 3
  2. Fish & Shrimps 5
  3. Spices 5
B. The AilamA® Cookbook Recommends 6
C. The AilamA® Cookbook Recommends 7
D. The AilamA® Emotional Cookbook 8
The AilamA® Recipes
WEEK 1
Alga Frittata 11
  You Matter! 13
Tuna Dipping Sauce 14
  You Matter! 16
WEEK 2
Bean Noodles Yum 17
  You Matter! 20
WEEK 3
Quinoa Wok Veggie 21
  You Matter! 24
Homemade Kefir 25
  You Matter! 27
WEEK 4
Royal Wok 28
  You Matter! 31
Caro-Coffee 32
  You Matter! 34
WEEK 5
Homemade Pressed Cheese 35
  You Matter! 37
Whey Pancakes 38
  You Matter! 40

WEEK 6

Smartly Dressed Salad 41

    You Matter! 43

WEEK 7

Meaty Soup 44

    You Matter! 46

WEEK 8

Millet Pudding 47

    You Matter! 49

Caro-Cream 50

    You Matter! 52

WEEK 9

Cranberry Salad 53

    You Matter! 55

WEEK 10

Pickled Horseradish 56

    You Matter! 58

Big Sushi 59

    You Matter! 62

WEEK 11

Bread Booster 63

    You Matter! 65

Fluffy Cake 66

    You Matter! 68

WEEK 12

Choco-Nut 69

    You Matter! 71

Homemade Yogurt 72

    You Matter! 74

WEEK 13

Parsley Salad 75

    You Matter! 77

Fig Truffles 78

    You Matter! 80

WEEK 14

Patties 81

    You Matter! 84

Milk Thistle Crunch 85

    You Matter! 87

WEEK 15
Choco Cake … 88
  You Matter! … 91
Veg-Sushi … 92
  You Matter! … 94
WEEK 16
Berry Cake … 95
  You Matter! … 97
Cocktail Skewers … 98
  You Matter! … 100
WEEK 17
Homemade Pâté … 101
  You Matter! … 103
 Butter Fruit Cocktail … 104
  You Matter! … 106
WEEK 18
Sweet-Sour Chicken … 107
  You Matter! … 109
Truffles Chameleon … 110
  You Matter! … 112
WEEK 19
Leek Wok … 113
  You Matter! … 115
WEEK 20
Broccoli Wok … 116
  You Matter! … 118
WEEK 21
China Mix … 119
  You Matter! … 121
WEEK 22
Minty Brown Cream … 122
  You Matter! … 124
Potato & Mushroom Stew … 125
  You Matter! … 127
WEEK 23
Choco-Delight … 128
  You Matter! … 130
Veggie Stew … 131
  You Matter! … 133

WEEK 24

Baked Meat — 134
  You Matter! — 136
Cedar Nut Dressing — 137
  You Matter! — 139

WEEK 25

Seaweed Salad — 140
  You Matter! — 142
Ruby Sour-Sweet — 143
  You Matter! — 145

WEEK 26

Choco-Exotique — 146
  You Matter! — 148
O-Sushi — 149
  You Matter! — 151

WEEK 27

Rice Boost — 152
  You Matter! — 154
Honey-Delight — 155
  You Matter! — 157

WEEK 28

Veggie White Delight — 158
  You Matter! — 161
Baked Squash — 162
  You Matter! — 164

WEEK 29

Old Sushi — 165
  You Matter! — 167
Baked Quince — 168
  You Matter! — 170

WEEK 30

Dinkel Flatties — 171
  You Matter! — 173
Sweet-Sour Comfy — 174
  You Matter! — 176

WEEK 31

Mashed Black Bean — 177
  You Matter! — 179

Chicory Sweet-Eyed Cookies ... 180
   You Matter! ... 182

WEEK 32
Brocco White Delight ... 183
   You Matter! ... 185
Plum Yum-Yum ... 186
   You Matter! ... 188

WEEK 33
Broil & Bake Salad ... 189
   You Matter! ... 191
Caramel Pudding ... 192
   You Matter! ... 194

WEEK 34
Cheerful Wok ... 195
   You Matter! ... 197
Pickled Cucumbers ... 198
   You Matter! ... 200

WEEK 35
Stir Fried Eggplants ... 201
   You Matter! ... 203
Cinnamon Spice Sweet ... 204
   You Matter! ... 206

WEEK 36
Sweet Potato Salad ... 207
   You Matter! ... 209
Squash Cake ... 210
   You Matter! ... 212

WEEK 37
Cabbage Wok ... 213
   You Matter! ... 215

WEEK 38
Kefir Cheese ... 216
   You Matter! ... 218
K-Sushi ... 219
   You Matter! ... 221

WEEK 39
Wok Delight ... 222
   You Matter! ... 224

Raspberry Cake 225
   You Matter! 227

WEEK 40
Mixed Salad 228
   You Matter! 230

WEEK 41
Pizza Chameleon 231
   You Matter! 234
Chico-Tea 235
   You Matter! 237

WEEK 42
Macrobiotic Soup 238
   You Matter! 240

WEEK 43
Minced Mix 241
   You Matter! 243
Baked Apples 244
   You Matter! 246

WEEK 44
Red Pepper Dipping Sauce 247
   You Matter! 249

WEEK 45
Prune Cake 250
   You Matter! 252
Dandelion-Root Coffee 253
   You Matter! 255

WEEK 46
T-Sushi 256
   You Matter! 258

WEEK 47
Veggie Cream 259
   You Matter! 262

WEEK 48
Salmon-Chicken Salad 263
   You Matter! 265
Chocolate Sweet Delight 266
   You Matter! 269

WEEK 49
Coco Cold 270
  You Matter! 272
Thy Stew 273
  You Matter! 276
WEEK 50
Mashed Parsnips 277
  You Matter! 279
WEEK 51
Buckwheat Salad 280
  You Matter! 282
WEEK 52
Homemade Mozzarella 283
  You Matter! 285
Almond Cake 286
  You Matter! 288
The AilamA® Special Recipes
Happy Oils 289
  You Matter! 291
Happy Hair 292
  You Matter! 294
About The AilamA® Nutrition Program 296
The AilamA® 28-Day Nutrition Program
Days 1-2 297
Days 3-4 298
Days 5-6 299
Days 7-8 300
Days 9-10 301
Days 11-12 302
Days 13-14 303
Days 15-16 304
Days 17-18 305
Days 19-20 306
Days 21-22 307
Days 23-24 308
Days 25-26 309
Days 27-28 310

The AilamA® Nutrition Program Q&A

Is The AilamA® Nutrition Program specially designed for me? — 312

Can The AilamA® Nutrition Program provide the necessary nutrients
for both sedentary and physically active people? — 312

Can The AilamA® Nutrition Program be a weight-loss program? — 312

Should I eat less food a day if I want to lose weight? — 315

What if I get bored with The AilamA® Nutrition Program? — 315

How do I know how many carbs to eat daily? — 316

How much water should I drink daily? — 316

Why do I lose weight very quickly only in the first weeks? — 317

How does the principle of burning more calories than you eat apply
to people who are genetically predisposed to being either thin or obese? — 318

Should I eat snacks during the day? — 318

Should I be taking supplements? — 319

Can The AilamA® Nutrition Program help me get rid of cellulite? — 319

Should I use only organic ingredients when cooking the dishes included
in The AilamA® Nutrition Program? — 320

Can I use The AilamA® Nutrition Program for longer than a week,
if I feel it's beneficial to me? — 320

How can I tailor The AilamA® Nutrition Program to my own needs,
if I want to stick with it? — 321

Can The AilamA® Nutrition Program help me overcome emotional eating? — 321

What else should I know before embarking on The AilamA®
Nutrition Program? — 323

The AilamA® Recipes

SOUPS

Meaty Soup … 44
Macrobiotic Soup … 238
Veggie Cream … 259

WOKS

Bean Noodles Yum … 17
Quinoa Wok Veggie … 21
Royal Wok … 28
Sweet-Sour Chicken … 107
Leek Wok … 113
Broccoli Wok … 116
China Mix … 119
Cheerful Wok … 195
Stir Fried Eggplants … 201
Cabbage Wok … 213
Wok Delight … 222

OMELETS

Alga Frittata … 11

MEATS

Cocktail Skewers … 98
Baked Meat … 134
Minced Mix … 241

STEWS

Potato & Mushroom Stew … 125
Veggie Stew … 131
Veggie White Delight … 158
Brocco White Delight … 183
Thy Stew … 273

DAIRY

Homemade Kefir … 25
Homemade Pressed Cheese … 35
Homemade Yogurt … 72
Kefir Cheese … 216
Homemade Mozzarella … 283

SALADS

Smartly Dressed Salad … 41
Cranberry Salad … 53

Parsley Salad	75
Seaweed Salad	140
Broil & Bake Salad	189
Sweet Potato Salad	207
Mixed Salad	228
Salmon-Chicken Salad	263
Buckwheat Salad	280

SAUCES

Tuna Dipping Sauce	14
Cheddar Nut Dressing	137
Red Pepper Dipping Sauce	247

SPREADS

Homemade Pâté	101
Mashed Black Bean	177
Mashed Parsnips	277

BREAD

| Bread Booster | 63 |
| Dinkel Flatties | 171 |

PICKLES

| Pickled Horseradish | 56 |
| Pickled Cucumbers | 198 |

PIZZA

| Pizza Chameleon | 231 |

SUSHI

Big Sushi	59
Veg-Sushi	92
O-Sushi	149
Old Sushi	165
K-Sushi	219
T-Sushi	256

GRAINS

| Millet Pudding | 47 |
| Rice Boost | 152 |

BEVERAGES

Caro-Coffee	32
Milk Thistle Crunch	85
Chico-Tea	235
Dandelion-Root Coffee	253

CAKES

Whey Pancakes	38
Fluffy Cake	66
Choco Cake	88
Berry Cake	95
Sweet-Sour Comfy	174
Squash Cake	210
Raspberry Cake	225
Prune Cake	250
Chocolate Sweet Delight	266
Almond Cake	286

COOKIES

Patties	81
Chicory Sweet-Eyed Cookies	180
Cinnamon Spice Sweet	204

TRUFFLES

Fig Truffles	78
Truffles Chameleon	110

CREAMS

Caro-Cream	50
Choco-Nut	69
Minty Brown Cream	122
Choco-Delight	128
Choco Exotique	146
Honey-Delight	155
Caramel Pudding	192

PRESERVES & JAMS

Ruby Sour-Sweet	143
Plum Yum-Yum	186

FRUIT

Butter Fruit Cocktail	104
Baked Squash	162
Baked Quince	168
Baked Apples	244

ICE CREAM

Coco Cold	270

SPECIALS

Happy Oils	289
Happy Hair	292

The AilamA® Emotional Cookbook

WEEK 1
Fear: Alga Frittata — 11
Anger: Tuna Dipping Sauce — 14
WEEK 2
Sadness: Bean Noodles Yum — 17
WEEK 3
Joy: Quinoa Wok Veggie — 21
Pessimism: Homemade Kefir — 25
WEEK 4
Surprise: Royal Wok — 28
Craving: Caro-Coffee — 32
WEEK 5
Determination: Homemade Pressed Cheese — 35
Acceptance: Whey Pancakes — 38
WEEK 6
Allowing: Smartly Dressed Salad — 41
WEEK 7
Admiration: Meaty Soup — 44
WEEK 8
Lack of Motivation: Millet Pudding — 47
Relaxation: Caro-Cream — 50
WEEK 9
Anticipation: Cranberry Salad — 53
WEEK 10
Confidence: Pickled Horseradish — 56
Loyalty: Big Sushi — 59
WEEK 11
Gratitude: Bread Booster — 63
Invincibility: Fluffy Cake — 66
WEEK 12
Ambition: Choco-Nut — 69
Romantic Boredom: Homemade Yogurt — 72
WEEK 13
Courage: Parsley Salad — 75
Overexcitement & Insecurity: Fig Truffles — 78

WEEK 14

Lack of Overreaction: Patties 81

Comfort & Joy: Milk Thistle Crunch 85

WEEK 15

Love: Choco Cake 88

Longing: Veg-Sushi 92

WEEK 16

Motivation: Berry Cake 95

Pleasure: Cocktail Skewers 98

WEEK 17

Nostalgia: Homemade Pâté 101

Shame: Butter Fruit Cocktail 104

WEEK 18

Disappointment: Sweet-Sour Chicken 107

Worries: Truffles Chameleon 110

WEEK 19

Comfort: Leek Wok 113

WEEK 20

Kindness: Broccoli Wok 116

WEEK 21

Harmony: China Mix 119

WEEK 22

Sympathy: Minty Brown Cream 122

Anger: Potato & Mushroom Stew 125

WEEK 23

Suffering: Choco-Delight 128

Courage: Veggie Stew 131

WEEK 24

Jealousy: Baked Meat 134

Loneliness: Cedar Nut Dressing 137

WEEK 25

Confidence: Seaweed Salad 140

Loneliness: Ruby Sour-Sweet 143

WEEK 26

Confidence: Choco-Exotique 146

Restlessness: O-Sushi 149

WEEK 27

Energy: Rice Boost 152

Lack of Appreciation: Honey-Delight 155

WEEK 28

Sociability: *Veggie White Delight* ... 158

Anxiety: *Baked Squash* ... 162

WEEK 29

Convenience: *Old Sushi* ... 165

Weep: *Baked Quince* ... 168

WEEK 30

Exhaustion: *Dinkel Flatties* ... 171

Balance: *Sweet-Sour Comfy* ... 174

WEEK 31

Criticism: *Mashed Black Bean* ... 177

Relaxation: *Chicory Sweet-Eyed Cookies* ... 180

WEEK 32

Fear & Unease: *Brocco White Delight* ... 183

Self-Doubt & Denial: *Plum Yum-Yum* ... 186

WEEK 33

Sadness: *Broil & Bake Salad* ... 189

Courage: *Caramel Pudding* ... 192

WEEK 34

Determination: *Cheerful Wok* ... 195

Equilibrium: *Pickled Cucumbers* ... 198

WEEK 35

Celebration: *Stir Fried Eggplants* ... 201

Craving: *Cinnamon Spice Sweet* ... 204

WEEK 36

Love: *Sweet Potato Salad* ... 207

Preoccupation: *Squash Cake* ... 210

WEEK 37

Helplessness: *Cabbage Wok* ... 213

WEEK 38

Creativity: *Kefir Cheese* ... 216

Devotion: *K-Sushi* ... 219

WEEK 39

Reflection: *Wok Delight* ... 222

Femininity: *Raspberry Cake* ... 225

WEEK 40

Guilt: *Mixed Salad* ... 228

WEEK 41

Nostalgia: *Pizza Chameleon* ... 231

Enthusiasm: *Chico-Tea* ... 235

WEEK 42

Satisfaction: Macrobiotic Soup — 238

WEEK 43

Satisfaction: Minced Mix — 241

Loneliness: Baked Apples — 244

WEEK 44

Tiredness & Self-Dislike: Red Pepper Dipping Sauce — 247

WEEK 45

Relaxation: Prune Cake — 250

Tiredness: Dandelion-Root Coffee — 253

WEEK 46

Care: T-Sushi — 256

WEEK 47

Relaxation: Veggie Cream — 259

WEEK 48

Weep: Salmon-Chicken Salad — 263

Depression & Confusion: Chocolate Sweet Delight — 266

WEEK 49

Boredom: Coco Cold — 270

Sadness: Thy Stew — 273

WEEK 50

Happiness: Mashed Parsnips — 277

WEEK 51

Consistency: Buckwheat Salad — 280

WEEK 52

Satisfaction: Homemade Mozzarella — 283

Craving: Almond Cake — 286

The AilamA® Emotional Index

Acceptance: Whey Pancakes — 38
Admiration: Meaty Soup — 44
Allowing: Smartly Dressed Salad — 41
Ambition: Choco-Nut — 69
Anger: Tuna Dipping Sauce — 14
    Potato & Mushroom Stew — 125
Anticipation: Cranberry Salad — 53
Anxiety: Baked Squash — 162
Balance: Sweet-Sour Comfy — 174
Boredom: Coco Cold — 270
    Homemade Yogurt — 72
Care: T-Sushi — 256
Celebration: Stir Fried Eggplants — 201
Comfort: Milk Thistle Crunch — 85
    Leek Wok — 113
Confidence: Pickled Horseradish — 56
    Seaweed Salad — 140
    Choco-Exotique — 146
Confusion: Chocolate Sweet Delight — 266
Consistency: Buckwheat Salad — 280
Convenience: Old Sushi — 165
Courage: Parsley Salad — 75
    Veggie Stew — 131
    Caramel Pudding — 192
Craving: Caro-Coffee — 32
    Cinnamon Spice Sweet — 204
    Almond Cake — 286
Creativity: Kefir Cheese — 216
Criticism: Mashed Black Bean — 177
Denial: Plum Yum-Yum — 186
Depression: Chocolate Sweet Delight — 266
Determination: Homemade Pressed Cheese — 35
    Cheerful Wok — 195
Devotion: K-Sushi — 219
Disappointment: Sweet-Sour Chicken — 107

Energy: Rice Boost   152
Enthusiasm: Chico-Tea   235
Equilibrium: Pickled Cucumbers   198
Exhaustion: Dinkel Flatties   171
Fear: Alga Frittata   11
       Brocco White Delight   183
Femininity: Raspberry Cake   225
Gratitude: Bread Booster   63
Guilt: Mixed Salad   228
Happiness: Mashed Parsnips   277
Harmony: China Mix   119
Helplessness: Cabbage Wok   213
Insecurity: Fig Truffles   78
Invincibility: Fluffy Cake   66
Jealousy: Baked Meat   134
Joy: Quinoa Wok Veggie   21
       Milk Thistle Crunch   85
Kindness: Broccoli Wok   116
Lack of Appreciation: Honey-Delight   155
Lack of Motivation: Millet Pudding   47
Lack of Overreaction: Patties   81
Loneliness: Cedar Nut Dressing   137
       Ruby Sour-Sweet   143
       Baked Apples   244
Longing: Veg-Sushi   92
Love: Choco Cake   88
       Sweet Potato Salad   207
Loyalty: Big Sushi   59
Motivation: Berry Cake   95
Nostalgia: Homemade Pâté   101
       Pizza Chameleon   231
Overexcitement: Fig Truffles   78
Pessimism: Homemade Kefir   25
Pleasure: Cocktail Skewers   98
Preoccupation: Squash Cake   210
Reflection: Wok Delight   222

Relaxation: Caro-Cream   50
       Chicory Sweet-Eyed Cookies   180
       Prune Cake   250
       Veggie Cream   259
Restlessness: O-Sushi   149
Sadness: Bean Noodles Yum   17
       Broil & Bake Salad   189
       Thy Stew   273
Satisfaction: Macrobiotic Soup   238
       Minced Mix   241
       Homemade Mozzarella   283
Self-Dislike: Red Pepper Dipping Sauce   247
Self-Doubt: Plum Yum-Yum   186
Shame: Butter Fruit Cocktail   104
Sociability: Veggie White Delight   158
Suffering: Choco-Delight   128
Surprise: Royal Wok   28
Sympathy: Minty Brown Cream   122
Tiredness: Red Pepper Dipping Sauce   247
       Dandelion-Root Coffee   253
Unease: Brocco White Delight   183
Weep: Baked Quince   168
       Salmon-Chicken Salad   263
Worries: Truffles Chameleon   110

Introduction

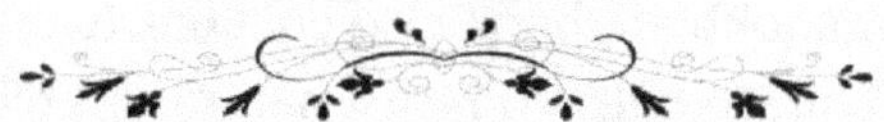

Hello, dear truth seeker!

How is your tri-faceted self feeling today?

Thank you for learning new things every day about yourself and the world we live in! And thank you for protecting our beloved planet by being your true self!

You are reading these lines because you want to be healthy, happy, and fulfilled at all times, and therefore healthy eating is definitely one of the cornerstones of your harmony and balance.

Naturally, your way of cooking combines all the nutrition information you have been garnering for years, consciously and unconsciously. That's a significant part of how you are evolving and keeping your body healthy. But you are well aware that the synergy of your body, mind, and soul can be easily disturbed by any dysfunction, big or small.

That's why you should trust your own individuality before anything else! It's the only way to remain connected to the universal truths stored within your subconscious mind from the very beginning of your life on Earth. One of these truths says that there is only health in the Universal Substance, whose perfect part you are right now!

You certainly know that there's no such thing as a completely new recipe. The ingredients are always the same precious gifts offered by our beloved planet, but we can anytime add a magic touch to a traditional recipe through different cooking methods and/or surprising combinations.

You may also know that it's more about how we eat than what we eat, and that one man's food may be someone else's poison.

Always listen to your body's signals! If you are told, for instance, that a certain vegetable is miraculous, but your body rejects it, don't struggle to push a square peg into a round hole.

If you still wonder why we are all craving highly processed foods, please remember that the act of healthy dieting starts in the mind, as does anything else. In time, our minds can better differentiate between detrimental and beneficial foods on more grounds than just taste and smell, especially when our liver and gallbladder start to function properly.

The AilamA® Cookbook is primarily a 365 culinary project, but also a comprehensive personal guide to emotional eating, a 28-day eating plan, and, last but not least, a very special English-learning textbook.

There are fifty-two weeks in a year. You can start this 365-day culinary journey at any time. Read the two recipes of each week and feel free to adjust them to your uniqueness (sometimes, there is only one recipe per week).You can even put the weeks and their corresponding recipes in a different order, if that's what you feel like doing.

As an added bonus, this cookbook book also contains two special recipes, one for your skin, the other for your hair, to help you trust natural ingredients even more.

On the interactive pages *You Matter*!, you can write down your sincere answers to the questions related to the proposed recipes.

Make sure you take the most artistic pictures you can of the foods you have cooked following The AilamA® Recipes.

Since The AilamA® Cookbook is much more than a 365 project, it can also help you make peace with your emotional eating through an overt relation between The AilamA® Recipes and no less than seventy of your main feelings. As an added bonus, there is a table of contents for The AilamA® Emotional Cookbook and a list of your positive and negative emotions in alphabetical order, called The AilamA® Emotional Index.

The AilamA® Nutrition Program is a 28-day meal plan based on The AilamA® Recipes. It respects the general nutrition guidelines you can find in any reliable specialty book, yet without asking you to focus on endless calculations of calories or on exact percentages of nutrients such as proteins, carbohydrates, fats, vitamins, and minerals.

Unless you are in desperate need of a dramatic dietary change on grounds of poor health, in which case you should consult a local professional, The AilamA® Nutrition Program can provide you with a different view on your eating routines.

Because of the small quantities needed at each meal, this eating plan is perfect for the whole family so that you won't have to cook different dishes for others, but share the same meal with them, meat or no meat.

If your body responds well to The AilamA® Nutrition Program, you are free to prolong it indefinitely; or you can make any new combinations you want based on the dietary suggestions written before The AilamA® Recipes, or the answers to the dietary questions you will find right after The AilamA® Nutrition Program.

Whether you are a language learner and want to practice your English in a fun way, or you are a native speaker, The AilamA® Cookbook may be what you are looking for in order to preserve your greatness in the midst of your everyday life.

As to the specialized language, apart from the food vocabulary, The AilamA® Recipes also contain lots of imperative verbs, along with special adverbs and adverbial phrases, while they leave out most articles, pronouns, and connectives.

This multipurpose cooking journal is yours to work with in any way you like – just listen to your heart, the true captain of your body, mind, and soul!

Honor the act of cooking and eating while honoring your Yin and Yang energies! Your kitchen is your castle. Your food is your loyal, colorful servant. Be the queen or the king of your life! Eat healthily, exercise, meditate, think big!

You really matter! Cook, serve, enjoy!

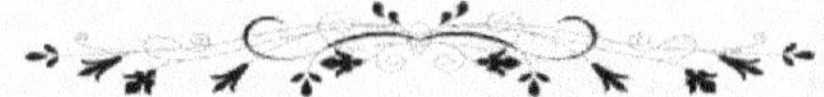

The AilamA® Cookbook is primarily offering quick and healthy recipes, whether you are a vegetarian or a meat-eater.

In a family, it should be easy to respect each other's dietary choices, right?

We should never eat anything detrimental for the mere reason that we have to cook for the whole family.

All the family chefs might be frowning now, thinking that The AilamA® Cookbook is going to advise them to prepare different, time-consuming dishes for each and every family member.

No way! The AilamA® Cookbook is going to ask nobody to spend the rest of their lives in the kitchen.

Instead, what about quick single-dish meals with different touches to please everyone?

A. The AilamA® Cookbook Recommends

1. Meat

You can always prepare meat separately from the rest of any dish.

Surprisingly enough, your meals will not be deprived of their meaty taste. On the contrary, they will abound in blending flavors.

Most importantly, they will be much healthier and will respect all the individualities sitting around the same table.

You can cook various types of meat in different ways, depending on their initial texture.

You should go for lean, fat-free organic meat, which comes from grass-fed animals, especially if you are a regular meat-eater. Thus, you will avoid ingesting considerable amounts of harmful hormones, or other dangerous chemical ingredients, along with your daily meals.

After having cooked meat in one of the ways mentioned below, you can cut it into small pieces, or grind it, in order to add it to your dishes.

The AilamA® Cookbook recommends that you cook meat before grinding it, instead of grinding it raw, especially when you use it in wok combinations.

Types of white & red meat

❖ **Organic poultry**

▪ chicken, hen, duck, turkey, rooster *(US)*/cock *(UK)*

❖ **Organic meat**

▪ veal, beef, lamb, mutton, venison, rabbit, hare

Types of cooking
❖ **Boiling**

   You can boil beef and venison.
1. Boil red meat slowly, for at least 30 minutes, in enough water to cover it.
2. Take all the scum away during the boiling process.
3. Take meat out and rinse it thoroughly in cold water.
4. Empty boiling water from the pot in order to wash it up, or use a different pot for the next step.
5. Put half-boiled meat in the pot again and cover it with fresh spring water.
6. Add condiments and continue to boil it for other 30-45 minutes.
7. Add salt 15 minutes prior to turning off the heat.

   You can use the remaining liquid as a stock for sauces, soups, or broths, if it's not too hard on your digestion.

❖ **Broiling***(US)*/**Grilling***(UK)*

   You should broil white or red meat only for a few minutes. In order to get that healthy brown color, you can cut a larger chunk into very thin slices.

❖ **Pickling** *(US)*/**Corning** *(UK)*

1. In a large glass bowl, put a generous amount of salt together with the juice and grated zest of a lemon.
2. Pour a large amount of spring water to completely cover the chunk of meat ready to be pickled.
3. Add a moderate onion, cut into small pieces, two egg yolks, two tablespoons of rice oil, together with all the fresh and dried herbs you want for extra flavor.
4. Gently whisk the combination thus obtained so that all of the ingredients will be well blended.
5. Soak the piece of meat in the pickling solution.
6. Cover the bowl with a glass lid and put it in the refrigerator for 24 hours.
7. When it's done, take the meat out and prepare it as you wish.

   The result will definitely be a piece of tender, delicious meat just ready to be combined with whatever vegetables and fruit you will choose for your dishes – or with the ones The AilamA® Cookbook recommends.

❖ **Slow roast-steaming**

   It's important that you buy a two-piece unglazed clay baking pot for your steak to be healthier and toxin-free in the end.
1. Let the piece of meat soak in boiling water for a few minutes to remove bacteria and chemicals, thus making it healthily edible.
2. Take the piece out of the soaking pot and place it inside the bottom part of the clay pot.

3. Rub the piece of meat with all the condiments and seasonings you want.
4. Add salt and spring water to cover the piece halfway. Water will make even the toughest meat tender, since this type of baking uses the principles of both steaming and roasting. You can also add some fresh herbs to the water for extra flavor.
5. Put the lid on to cover the bottom part perfectly.
6. Place the pot in the oven at the lowest temperature.

You can use this method of slow-baking for all kinds of meat, including chicken, hen, rooster, and turkey.

The covered pot should be kept in the oven for 3 to 4 hours, depending on the initial texture of the meat.

You can use the remaining liquid as a stock base for other dishes, after having sieved it twice. *(See also page 134.)*

2. Fish & Shrimps *(US)/***Prawns***(UK)*

You can prepare fish and shrimps separately from the rest of any dish, the way you will do with the other types of meat.

Types of organic fish
- salmon, cod, mackerel, tuna, trout, herring, sardine, sturgeon

Types of cooking

❖ **Baking**

You can bake whole fish, seasoning it before putting it into the oven. The baking time depends on the type of fish.

❖ **Broiling**

You can broil fish fillets and shrimps with condiments and salt until brown and juicy.

❖ **Steaming**

You should steam fish chunks and shrimps only for a few minutes, depending on their initial texture.

❖ **Boiling**

You should normally boil shrimps for half an hour or so.

3. Spices

Spices are essential for meals. They bring tremendous benefits to your health, since they are widely recognized as metabolic regulators, yeast and fungi healers, and digestive helpers, apart from the great taste they can add to your dishes.

You can have a glass jar in which you can mix all the seasonings you have in the kitchen, a teaspoonful of each.

You can also store them separately, if you want to enhance the taste of a particular spice in a dish.

You can use fresh herbs as well. You can grow them in small plant pots yourself. If it's their season, you can buy them from supermarkets or, better yet, from open-air markets.

In winters, it's best to use dried spices, if you want to avoid buying, for instance, a bunch of fresh parsley that looks so healthy, when it's actually packed with chemicals and fertilizers.

Types of dried spices
- anise, cinnamon, clove, curry, garlic, ginger, bay leaf, turmeric, saffron, caraway, fenugreek, cardamom, cumin, bergamot
- unrefined sea salt, unrefined rock salt
- dill, rosemary, sage, coriander, mint, thyme, oregano, marjoram, basil, lovage, tarragon

Types of fresh spices
- parsley, dill, sage, basil, thyme, tarragon, rosemary, oregano, lovage, coriander

B. The AilamA® Cookbook Recommends

Relearn old eating principles to the benefit of your health as a whole, in case you have forgotten them along the way.

Here's a small reminder:

- ❖ You should eat in a sitting position to avoid putting extra pressure on your digestive system.
- ❖ You should keep silent while eating to prevent extra air from entering your stomach and intestines.
- ❖ You should avoid eating when stressed. Even the most perfect diet may turn into poison if feelings of anxiety and worry accompany your meals.
- ❖ You should avoid rising from the table during meals. If you have forgotten something, try to adjust your eating to what is currently in front of you, if there isn't anyone around to bring you the forgotten item. At first, you may find it hard to impose this table behavior on yourself, but the bright side is that you'll become less forgetful in time.
- ❖ Try to eat in a comfortably straight position. If you have been unconsciously eating with your body twisted leftward or rightward, just imagine a creamy substance struggling to run through a winding conduit – it finally gets stuck.

- ❖ Try to produce a lot of happy thoughts while eating, especially thoughts related to the food on your plate.
- ❖ Give sincere thanks to the animals that sacrificed their lives to make your meals healthy and nutritious.
- ❖ Feel grateful for all the subtle processes of making your meals perfect in all the ways.
- ❖ Kindly ask the Universe to bless everyone and everything involved in the process of bringing the food into your country as well as to your neighborhood supermarket.
- ❖ Try to do nothing else while eating. In time, you'll find that, if you look at your food and concentrate only on it, it really has a different taste. Please rethink even the idea of making your meals more pleasant with some good music. The mixed emotions triggered by the chosen songs may add unwanted tension to your body, mind, and soul. But you can always listen to 432 Hz music, whatever else you are doing. You may already know that listening to 432 Hz music releases our emotional blockages and expands our consciousness, creating unity instead of separation.

C. The AilamA® Cookbook Recommends

Be the creative type of chef. Feel free to add, subtract, or adjust the amount of ingredients whenever you try something new.

Don't be afraid *not* to read a new recipe till its end. If a keyword within it can make you go in a different direction, feel free to experiment with different ingredients to obtain something completely new in the end.

If you are not a calorie person, it's not a big deal. If we chose to quantify the amounts of carbohydrates, proteins, and fats every time we eat, we would gradually lose the ability to listen to the cellular voice of our harmonious beings. That *is* a big deal, since we will practically forget how to understand and respect our individualities.

You should know, of course, how to interpret the nutritional information written on food packages. Yet don't be obsessed with numbers and percentages when it comes to healthy eating.

If you listen to your body, you will want to use more often easy units of measurement, like your palms, as well as the cups, glasses, teaspoons, and tablespoons in your kitchen.

Also, trust your personal perception of what small, medium, and large means in terms of eye-weighing the ingredients or the bunches of greens to be used in recipes.

If you trust it implicitly, your intuition will merge so well with your five-sensory nature that you will naturally feel the right quantities of the recipe components or the perfect sizes of your dishes. In this way, your recipes will bring extra flavor each time you want to exert your universal right to change and evolve.

Don't eat too much at meals, preferably one course, but eat whenever you are hungry. If you are perfectly healthy, you should include nutrient-dense snacks in your nutrition program on a regular basis.

Always eat a proper breakfast consisting of healthy whole foods.

Avoid combining meat with grains or grain products such as bread or pasta.

You can cook fruit in different combinations, with vegetables and meat, but you can also eat raw fruit in the morning or have a fruit snack between breakfast and lunch, if you have enjoyed a hearty dinner the evening before.

Even if you are a meat-eater, your meals can consist mainly of vegetables and fruit, with meat simply added to them after it has been prepared separately.

Try to eat the last meal at least 1½ hours before bedtime, or even less, if you suffer from hyperacidity.

Try not to weigh or measure yourself too often. Your eyes and clothes should tell you all you need to know about which way your body is headed.

D. The AilamA® Emotional Cookbook

Basically, emotional eating can be regarded as hunger that should not exist driven by feelings that should be healed, but that does not mean that natural hunger cannot be a healthy form of emotional eating.

Avoiding everyday temptations may be the hardest decision of all in the attempt to maintain a healthy lifestyle or to improve the quality of life.

We should all be proud of ourselves when we resist eating junk food, since what we eat has a huge amount of influence over our endocrine system and consequently over our metabolism and physiological needs.

However, we are emotional beings, so it goes without saying that any eating behavior will invariably be triggered by or nourish certain moods.

So, if we choose certain foods to accompany our good or bad moods, it doesn't necessarily mean that we lack self-control or that we have a weak willpower.

Instead of denying our social nature, we should just try to diversify the methods of regulating our stress-triggered emotions while accepting, once and for all, that all foods can speak to our hormones and feelings.

Only by embracing all of our emotional states, will we be able to develop, in time, a healthy relationship with food.

Thus, you can definitely use The AilamA® Cookbook both as a 365 culinary project and as an emotional nutrition guide.

There will be celebratory dishes, sealing your positive emotions, and comforting dishes, which will help you cope with loneliness, boredom, sadness, self-dislike, self-doubt, tiredness, nostalgia, or fear.

Whether you are a seasoned gourmand or you just enjoy culinary challenges, feel free to let The AilamA® Recipes inspire, heal, and regulate your emotional metabolism.

Your emotional eating is just another way of showing the strengths and weaknesses of your beautiful physicality.

Meant as terrific digestive aids and trustworthy beauty keepers, The AilamA® Recipes could regulate your metabolism, enhance your health and wellness, and help you lose weight naturally while boosting your energy and fitness levels. They could also accompany, regulate, and/or enhance your everyday feelings, turning your emotional eating into a healthy habit.

Curious to try them?

Feel free to embark upon this fun culinary journey!

Before choosing or deciding, take your time! Then, whatever you have chosen or decided to do, also take your time!

Simple and unforced ways are always the best.

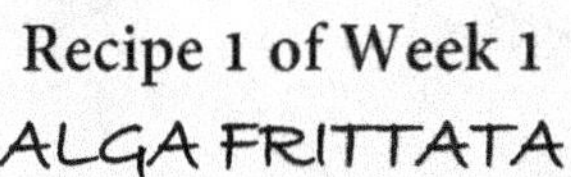

Recipe 1 of Week 1
ALGA FRITTATA

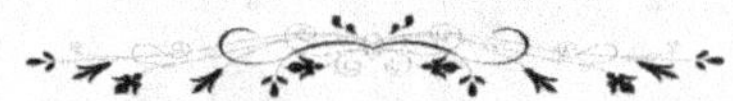

Here is a tasty dish with restorative properties to open your culinary project 365.

It can also be your comfort food when you are consciously afraid of something.

Always keep in mind that the only way out is through. Eat healthily and face your fears!

Type of meal	Breakfast Brunch Main Course
Type of Dish	Ovo-Vegetarian Non-Vegetarian
Preparation Time	Approximately 3 minutes Approximately 3 hours, soaking time
Cooking Time	Approximately 3 minutes
Servings	2
The AilamA® Cookbook advises You	You can make scrambled eggs by putting the mix, prepared as indicated below, into the pan and frequently stirring it until the eggs coagulate and form curds.

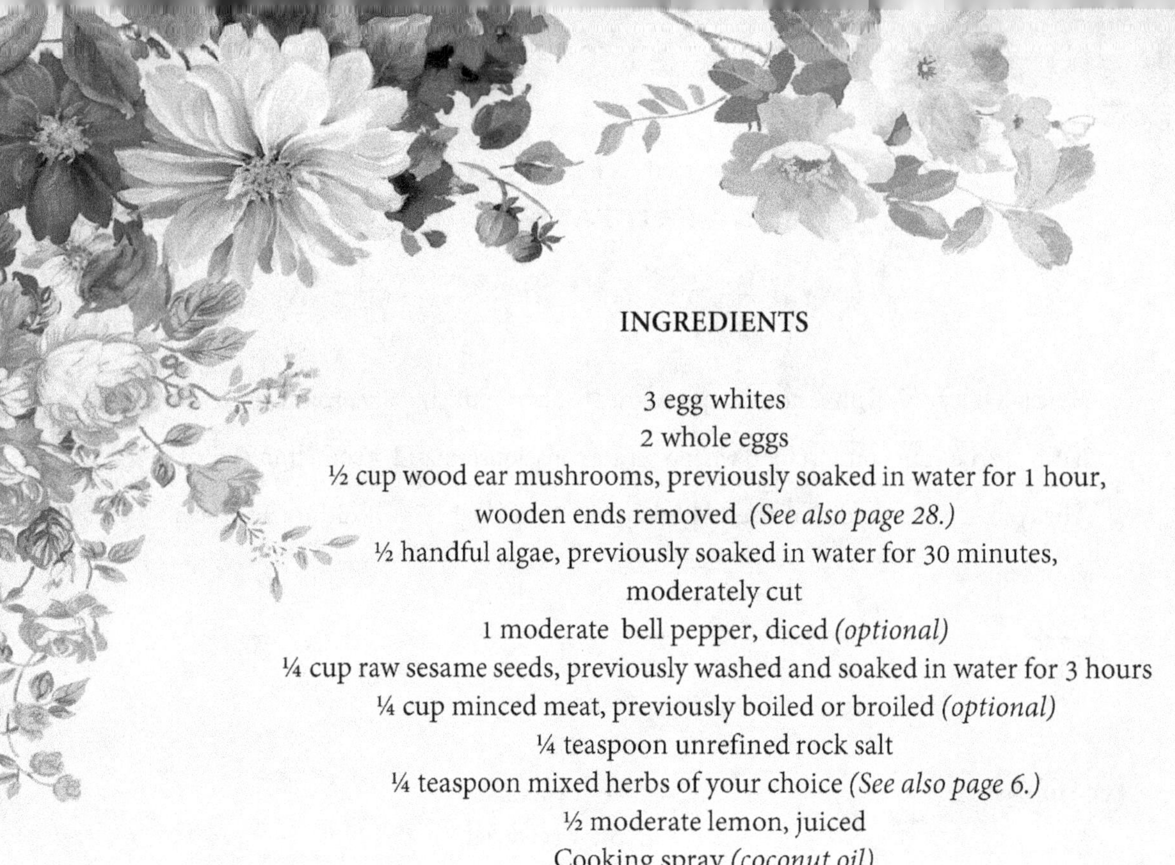

INGREDIENTS

3 egg whites
2 whole eggs
½ cup wood ear mushrooms, previously soaked in water for 1 hour,
wooden ends removed *(See also page 28.)*
½ handful algae, previously soaked in water for 30 minutes,
moderately cut
1 moderate bell pepper, diced *(optional)*
¼ cup raw sesame seeds, previously washed and soaked in water for 3 hours
¼ cup minced meat, previously boiled or broiled *(optional)*
¼ teaspoon unrefined rock salt
¼ teaspoon mixed herbs of your choice *(See also page 6.)*
½ moderate lemon, juiced
Cooking spray *(coconut oil)*

PREPARATION

1. Coat a medium non-stick frying pan with cooking spray.
2. Set pan over medium heat.
3. Whisk together eggs, egg whites, sesame seeds, meat, salt,
herbs, mushrooms, seaweed, and red pepper.
4. Put content into hot pan.
5. Let it cook.
6. Transfer to a large plate.
7. Slice in half for two servings.
8. Serve hot, warm, or at room temperature.

You Matter!

1. Take four gorgeous pictures of your culinary result.

2. Write down your impressions of the recipe.

a. Did you like it?

____

b. Was it difficult?

____

c. Did you find all the ingredients?

____

d. Did you make any changes to the recipe to better suit your dietary needs?

____

____

e. Will you cook it again?

____

f. Will you share it with your family and friends?

____

g. How did it make your body feel?

____

____

h. How were you feeling before cooking the recipe?

____

____

i. How were you feeling after eating the culinary result?

____

____

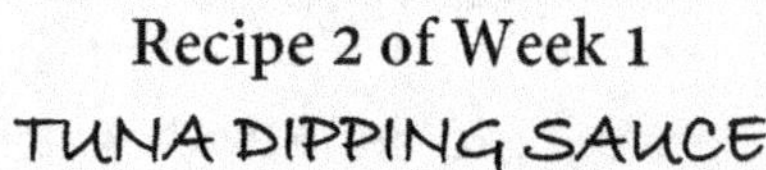

TUNA DIPPING SAUCE

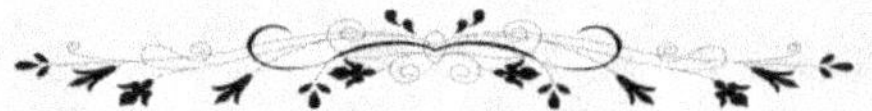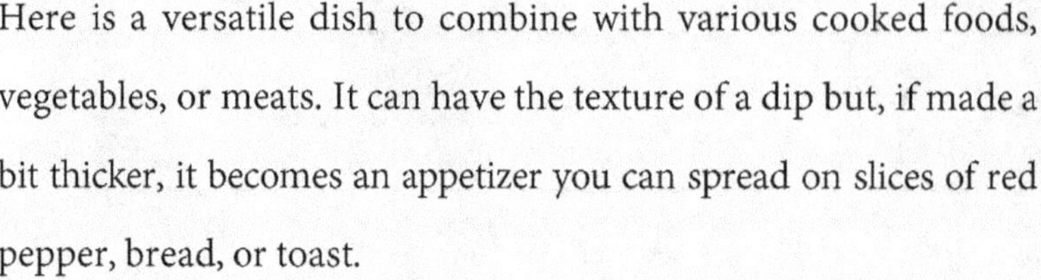

Here is a versatile dish to combine with various cooked foods, vegetables, or meats. It can have the texture of a dip but, if made a bit thicker, it becomes an appetizer you can spread on slices of red pepper, bread, or toast.

It can also help you ignore your anger when something has disturbed your peace of mind.

Type of Meal	Snack Breakfast
Type of Dish	Pesco-Vegetarian Non-Vegetarian
Preparation Time	Approximately 5 minutes
Cooking Time	Approximately 7 minutes, baking time
Servings	2 cups
The AilamA® Cookbook advises You	Soak canned tuna in cold spring water for 1 minute or so, and then rinse it thoroughly. This procedure will wash away the taste of staleness or canned fish.

INGREDIENTS

1 egg yolk
1 cup tuna fish, canned in brine
1 medium onion, previously baked
1 cup olive oil, extra virgin, unrefined
1 moderate lemon, juiced
1 cup spring water *(optional)*
1 tablespoon fresh parsley, washed and chopped
½ teaspoon mixed herbs of your choice *(See also page 6.)*

PREPARATION

1. Blend fish, oil, and lemon until smooth.
2. Add onion, salt, spices.
3. Blend until smooth.
4. Add water until desired consistency is achieved. *(optional)*
5. Transfer to a mixing bowl.
6. Add parsley.
7. Whisk it until desired smoothness is achieved.
8. Serve it chilled, with vegetables, salads, or meats.
9. Serve on slices of bread, toast, or red pepper.

You Matter!

1. Take four gorgeous pictures of your culinary result.

2. Write down your impressions of the recipe.

a. Did you like it?

____

b. Was it difficult?

____

c. Did you find all the ingredients?

____

d. Did you make any changes to the recipe to better suit your dietary needs?

____

____

e. Will you cook it again?

____

f. Will you share it with your family and friends?

____

g. How did it make your body feel?

____

____

h. How were you feeling before cooking the recipe?

____

____

i. How were you feeling after eating the culinary result?

____

____

The Recipe of Week 2
BEAN NOODLES YUM

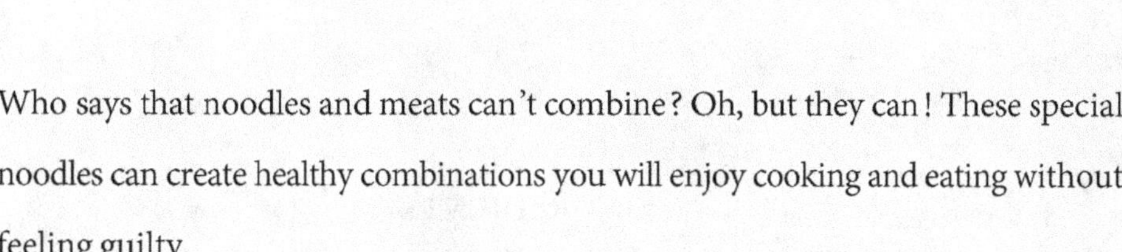

Who says that noodles and meats can't combine? Oh, but they can! These special noodles can create healthy combinations you will enjoy cooking and eating without feeling guilty.

You can also eat them whenever sadness is your sudden or unwanted companion.

Type of Meal	Main Course
	Lunch
	Dinner
Type of Dish	Vegetarian
	Ovo-Vegetarian
	Non-Vegetarian
Preparation Time	Approximately 5 minutes
	Approximately 1 hour, soaking time
Cooking Time	Approximately 10 minutes
Servings	4
The AilamA® Cookbook advises You	Bean noodles can definitely satisfy your craving for meat and starches at the same meal.

INGREDIENTS

1 pack bean thread noodles
1 large zucchini, moderately cut *(optional)*
1 large bell pepper, moderately cut
1 handful broccoli florets, halved *(optional)*
1 cup green peas, washed
2 celery stalks, moderately sliced *(optional)*
1 cup wood ear mushrooms, moderately cut,
previously soaked in water for 1 hour
1 red onion, moderately diced
3 cloves garlic, peeled and crushed
4 egg whites
3 tablespoons coconut oil
2 tablespoons pure dark sesame oil *(from roasted sesame seeds)*
2 teaspoons unrefined sea salt
1 teaspoon mixed herbs of your choice *(See also page 6.)*
Meat of your choice, minced or cut into bite-sized pieces,
after previously prepared as desired *(non-vegetarian dish)*

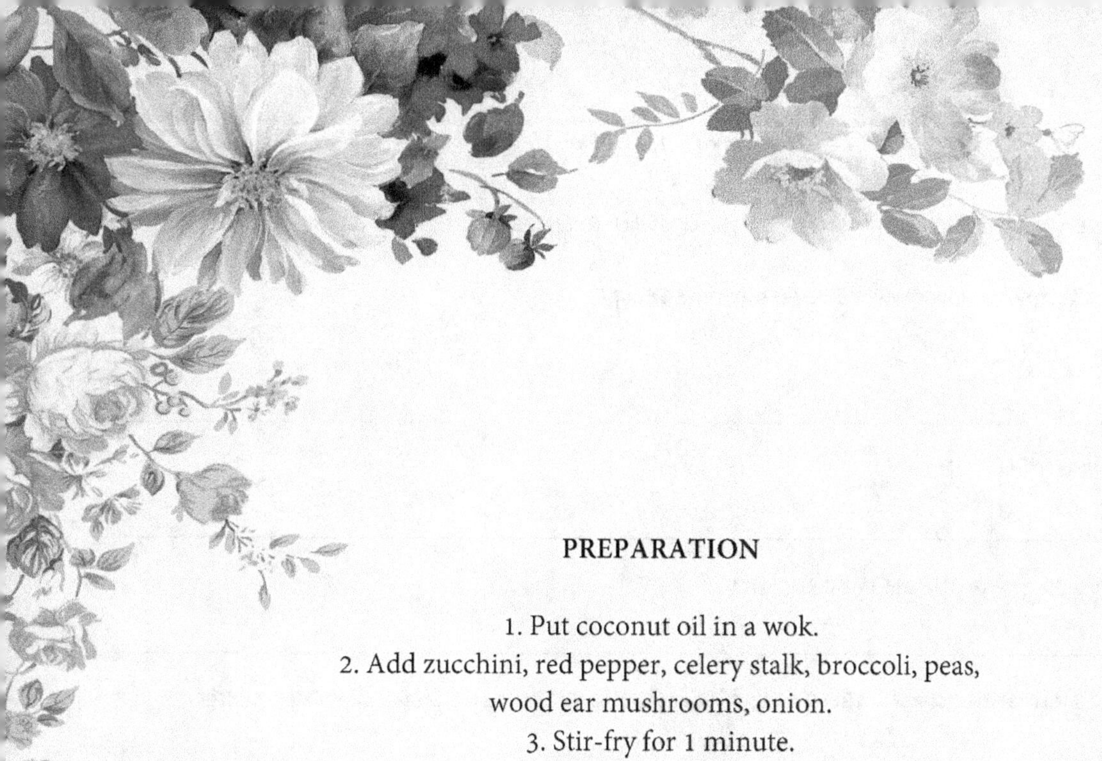

PREPARATION

1. Put coconut oil in a wok.
2. Add zucchini, red pepper, celery stalk, broccoli, peas, wood ear mushrooms, onion.
3. Stir-fry for 1 minute.
4. Add salt and herbs.
5. Stir-fry once again.
6. Let it cool for 1 minute.
7. Make scrambled egg whites.
8. Add scrambled egg whites to vegetables.
9. Add meat. *(non-vegetarian dish)*
10. Mix well.
11. Bring spring water to a boil.
12. Add 1 teaspoon sea salt.
13. Set it aside.
14. Add bean noodles.
15. Let them soak in lukewarm water for 12 minutes.
16. Transfer noodles to a large bowl.
17. Add wok mixture.
18. Stir until well combined.
19. Serve hot, warm, or cold.

You Matter!

1. Take four gorgeous pictures of your culinary result.

2. Write down your impressions of the recipe.

a. Did you like it?

____

b. Was it difficult?

____

c. Did you find all the ingredients?

____

d. Did you make any changes to the recipe to better suit your dietary needs?

____

____

e. Will you cook it again?

____

f. Will you share it with your family and friends?

____

g. How did it make your body feel?

____

____

h. How were you feeling before cooking the recipe?

____

____

i. How were you feeling after eating the culinary result?

____

____

QUINOA WOK VEGGIE

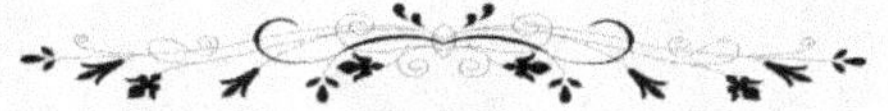

Quinoa with vegetables is a rich source of nutrients to help you keep healthy and fit, whether you are vegetarian or not.

It can also be your culinary companion whenever you feel lively and joyful.

Type of Meal	Main Course Lunch Dinner
Type of Dish	Vegetarian Ovo-Vegetarian Non-Vegetarian
Preparation Time	Approximately 10 minutes Approximately 1 hour, soaking time
Cooking Time	Approximately 10 minutes
Servings	4
The AilamA® Cookbook advises You	Let quinoa soak for at least 1 hour. Wash quinoa thoroughly before cooking it. Add spring water to cover it. Bring water to a boil, then reduce heat. Let content simmer until the liquid has boiled away. Add extra water if you consider that quinoa is not done. It should be creamy, not mushy. Quinoa can be found in health stores or in supermarkets. The organic type is preferable.

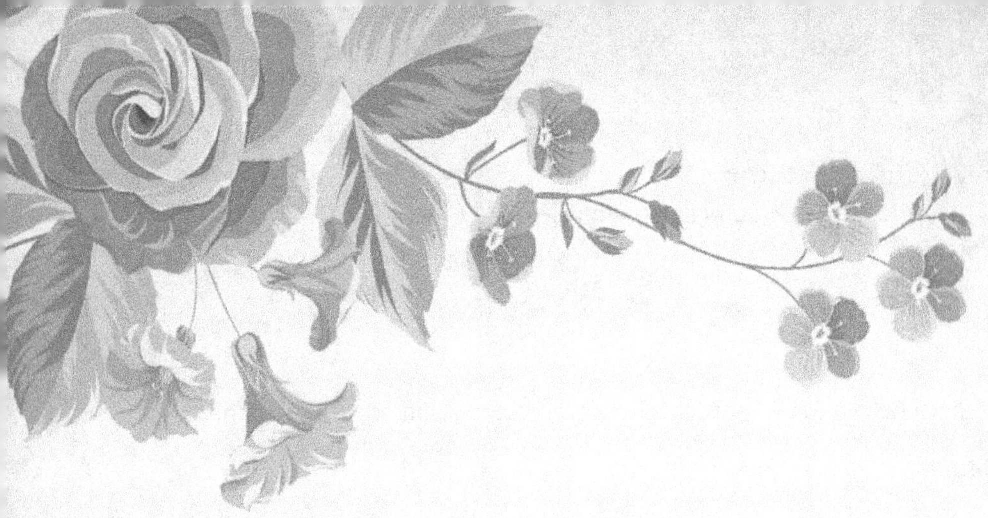

INGREDIENTS

2 large parsnips, cut into large chunks
½ medium celery root, cut into moderate chunks
2 medium bell peppers, sliced lengthwise then halved
1 medium carrot, sliced lengthwise then cut on the diagonal
2 medium zucchini, halved then cut into moderate chunks
2 tablespoons fresh parsley, including stems and roots, washed and chopped
2 tablespoons fresh dill, including stems and roots, washed and chopped
2 tablespoons fresh celery leaves, washed and chopped
2 celery stalks, washed and coarsely cut
2 medium onions, sliced in full rings
1 handful string beans, halved
4 egg whites
6 cloves garlic, chopped
1 teaspoon unrefined sea salt
3 tablespoons coconut oil
1 tablespoon pure sesame oil *(from roasted sesame seeds)*
2 teaspoons mixed herbs of your choice *(See also page 6.)*
2 handfuls quinoa

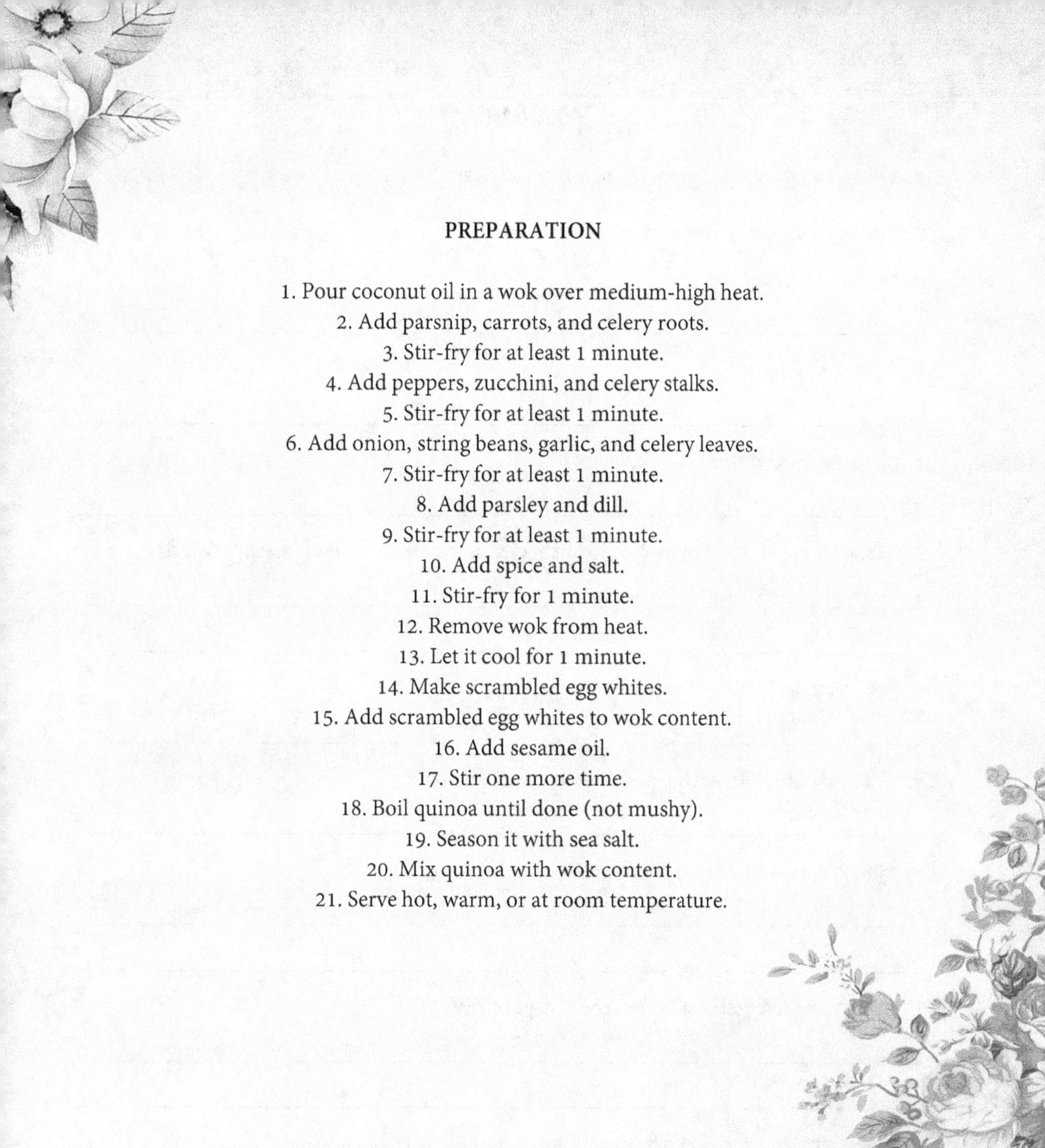

PREPARATION

1. Pour coconut oil in a wok over medium-high heat.
2. Add parsnip, carrots, and celery roots.
3. Stir-fry for at least 1 minute.
4. Add peppers, zucchini, and celery stalks.
5. Stir-fry for at least 1 minute.
6. Add onion, string beans, garlic, and celery leaves.
7. Stir-fry for at least 1 minute.
8. Add parsley and dill.
9. Stir-fry for at least 1 minute.
10. Add spice and salt.
11. Stir-fry for 1 minute.
12. Remove wok from heat.
13. Let it cool for 1 minute.
14. Make scrambled egg whites.
15. Add scrambled egg whites to wok content.
16. Add sesame oil.
17. Stir one more time.
18. Boil quinoa until done (not mushy).
19. Season it with sea salt.
20. Mix quinoa with wok content.
21. Serve hot, warm, or at room temperature.

You Matter!

1. Take four gorgeous pictures of your culinary result.

2. Write down your impressions of the recipe.

a. Did you like it?

____

b. Was it difficult?

____

c. Did you find all the ingredients?

____

d. Did you make any changes to the recipe to better suit your dietary needs?

____

____

e. Will you cook it again?

____

f. Will you share it with your family and friends?

____

g. How did it make your body feel?

____

____

h. How were you feeling before cooking the recipe?

____

____

i. How were you feeling after eating the culinary result?

____

____

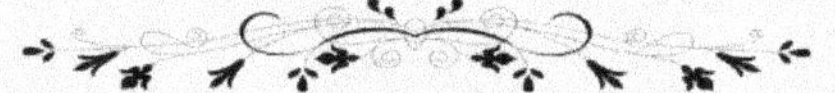

Here is the recipe for the healthiest lactose-free diary product, which can help redress many imbalances thanks to its many strains of good bacteria.

You can also drink this healthy beverage whenever you feel something is wrong with you or others – it could help you make more inspired decisions.

Type of Meal	Healthy Snack Appetizer
Type of Dish	Lacto-Vegetarian Non-Vegetarian
Preparation Time	Approximately 5 minutes
Cooking Time	Approximately 12-24 hours
Servings	8 cups
The AilamA® Cookbook advises You	In order to start your kefir journey, you can buy your first batch of kefir grains from a fellow kefir lover. Use only glass, plastic, and wooden utensils (no metal) when handling kefir grains. Using the same recipe, you can make coconut kefir from either coconut milk or coconut water. Make sure you alternate between milk and coconut so that the kefir grains have time to feed on milk. Or you can buy water kefir grains to culture sugar water, juice, or coconut water and milk.

INGREDIENTS

2 liters (~70 fl oz) skim milk *(bio)*
or
2 liters (~70 fl oz) whole milk *(bio)*
2 tablespoons kefir grains

PREPARATION

1. Pour milk over your kefir grains in a jar.
2. Cover jar with a plastic lid.
3. Let jar sit in a warm place, until kefir is cultured as desired (sour or sweeter).
4. Strain kefir.
5. Keep kefir in the refrigerator.
6. Place kefir grains into a new jar.
7. Pour new milk on top to start another batch.
8. Serve it with cereals, berries, homemade bread, or by itself.

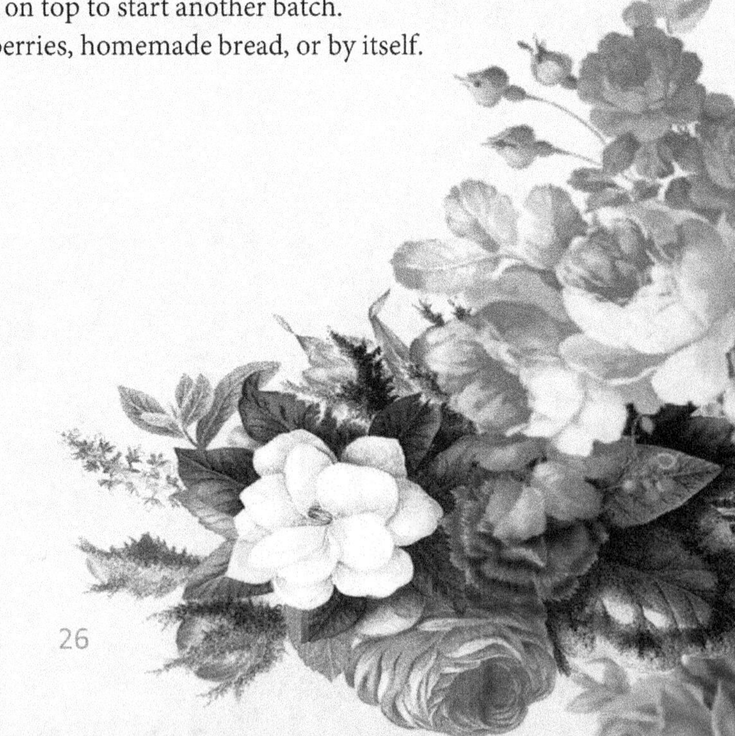

You Matter!

1. Take four gorgeous pictures of your culinary result.

2. Write down your impressions of the recipe.

a. Did you like it?

____

b. Was it difficult?

____

c. Did you find all the ingredients?

____

d. Did you make any changes to the recipe to better suit your dietary needs?

____

____

e. Will you cook it again?

____

f. Will you share it with your family and friends?

____

g. How did it make your body feel?

____

____

h. How were you feeling before cooking the recipe?

____

____

i. How were you feeling after eating the culinary result?

____

____

ROYAL WOK

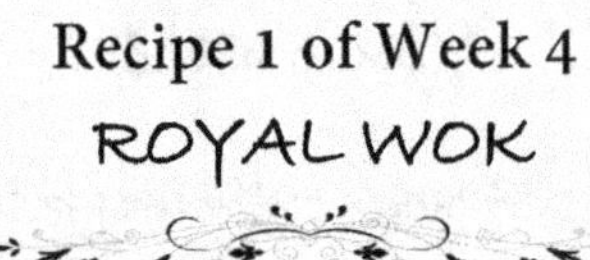
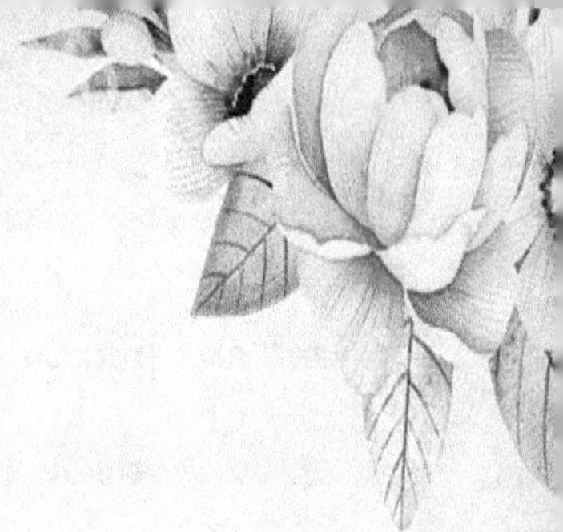

Not in love with wok vegetables yet? Here are some more combinations.
Also, it can be the perfect dish when something has taken you by surprise.

Type of Meal	Main Course
	Lunch
	Dinner
Type of Dish	Vegetarian
	Ovo-Vegetarian
	Non-Vegetarian
Preparation Time	Approximately 10 minutes
	Approximately 1 hour, soaking time
	Approximately 30 minutes, boiling time
Cooking Time	Approximately 10 minutes
Servings	4
The AilamA® Cookbook advises You	Wood ear mushrooms are usually sold dried, in medium-sized packs, but don't be deceived by their shrunken appearance. When in water, they become extremely large, so less than ¼ pack will normally do for woks and soups. Let them soak in warm spring water for about 1 hour. Next, wash and rinse them thoroughly, then cut off their wooden ends. Now, they are ready for any food combination you like.

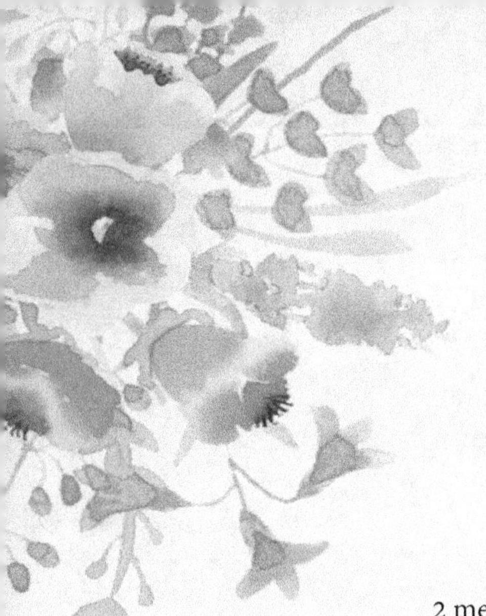

INGREDIENTS

2 medium bamboo shoots, thinly sliced
2 handfuls wood ear mushrooms
2 medium bell peppers, sliced lengthwise, then halved
¼ baked butternut pumpkin, cut into large chunks
3 tablespoons fresh celery leaves, washed and chopped
2 celery stalks, washed and coarsely cut
2 medium onions, sliced into full rings
1 handful string beans, previously halved and boiled
6 cloves garlic, chopped
4 egg whites
1 teaspoon unrefined sea salt
3 tablespoons coconut oil
1 tablespoon pure sesame oil *(from roasted sesame seeds)*
2 teaspoons mixed herbs of your choice *(See also page 6.)*
Chicken breast, minced or cut into bite-sized pieces,
after previously prepared as desired *(non-vegetarian dish)*

PREPARATION

1. Heat coconut oil in a wok over medium-high heat.
2. Add bamboo shoot, wood ear mushrooms,
string beans, celery stalks, and red peppers.
3. Stir-fry for at least 1 minute.
4. Add onion, garlic, and celery leaves.
5. Stir-fry for at least 1 minute.
6. Add baked pumpkin.
7. Stir-fry for at least 1 minute.
8. Add spice and salt.
9. Stir-fry for 1 minute.
10. Remove wok from heat.
11. Let it cool for 1 minute.
12. Make scrambled egg whites.
13. Add scrambled egg whites to wok content.
14. Add sesame oil.
15. Stir all ingredients one more time.
15. Add chicken breast. *(non-vegetarian dish)*
16. Stir one last time.
17. Serve hot, warm, or at room temperature.

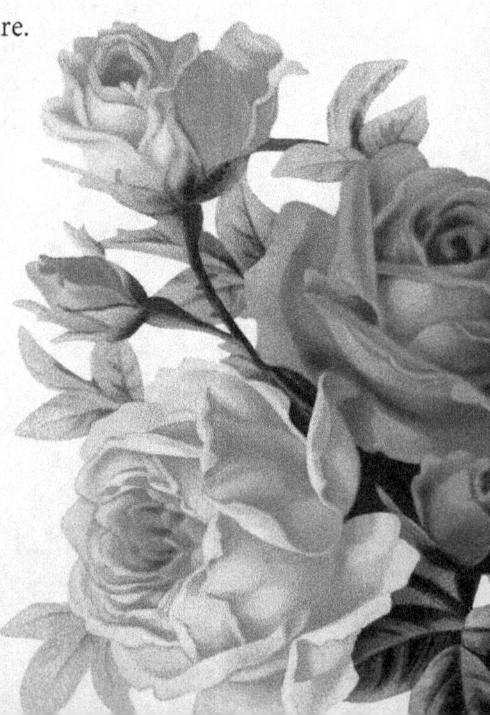

You Matter!

1. Take four gorgeous pictures of your culinary result.

2. Write down your impressions of the recipe.

a. Did you like it?

____

b. Was it difficult?

____

c. Did you find all the ingredients?

____

d. Did you make any changes to the recipe to better suit your dietary needs?

____

____

e. Will you cook it again?

____

f. Will you share it with your family and friends?

____

g. How did it make your body feel?

____

____

h. How were you feeling before cooking the recipe?

____

____

i. How were you feeling after eating the culinary result?

____

____

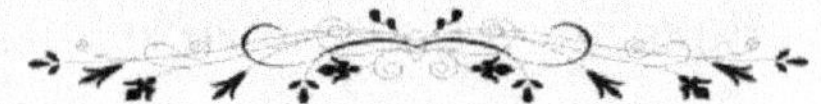

Good news, coffee lover! There are many healthy alternatives to the classic, caffeine-loaded mocha, and carob coffee is one of them.

You can also enjoy this versatile, naturally sweet beverage (with or without coconut milk) whenever you have a craving for hot chocolate.

Type of Meal	Snack
Type of Dish	Vegetarian Non-Vegetarian
Preparation Time	Approximately 3 minutes
Cooking Time	Approximately 10 minutes, roasting time for fresh carob pods Approximately 5 minutes, roasting time for dried carob pods Approximately 5 minutes, simmering time for carob powder Approximately 10 minutes, simmering time for carob pods
Servings	3 cups
The AilamA® Cookbook advises You	If you choose to make coffee from pod pieces instead of grinding them into powder, you can actually eat the pods after simmering them. However, chew them with great care, since there may still be some hard seeds left in the kibbles, and you don't want to break your teeth. *(See also page 50.)*

INGREDIENTS

1½ teaspoons carob powder, coarsely ground
or
2 tablespoons dried or roasted carob pod pieces, organic

PREPARATION

1. Bring 1¼ cups spring water to a boil.
2. Add 1½ teaspoons carob coffee or 2 tablespoons carob pods.
3. Simmer for 5 or 10 minutes.
4. Strain it through a fine mesh strainer.
5. Drink it hot, warm, or cold.
6. Drink it black.
7. Drink it with coconut milk. *(optional)*
8. Eat the boiled carob pods. *(optional)*
(See also pages 85 and 253.)

You Matter!

1. Take four gorgeous pictures of your culinary result.

2. Write down your impressions of the recipe.

a. Did you like it?

____

b. Was it difficult?

____

c. Did you find all the ingredients?

____

d. Did you make any changes to the recipe to better suit your dietary needs?

____

____

e. Will you cook it again?

____

f. Will you share it with your family and friends?

____

g. How did it make your body feel?

____

____

h. How were you feeling before cooking the recipe?

____

____

i. How were you feeling after eating the culinary result?

____

____

HOMEMADE PRESSED CHEESE

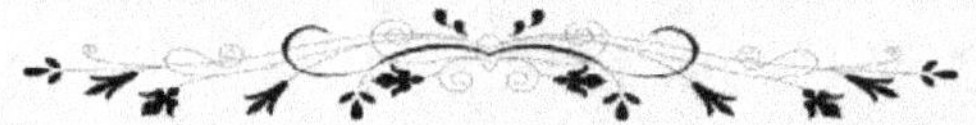

Here is the easiest recipe ever for pressed cheese. Make sure you use organic (bio) ingredients for optimum results.

You can also eat it when someone's choices or decisions inspired you with determination.

Type of Meal	Healthy Snack Appetizer
Type of Dish	Lacto-Vegetarian Non-Vegetarian
Preparation Time	Approximately 5 minutes
Cooking Time	Approximately 30 minutes
Servings	10
The AilamA® Cookbook advises You	It's up to you how much fat you want your pressed cheese to contain. If you want it quite fat, then you can opt for whole milk and cream with the highest fat content. If you want a low-fat version, then you can combine skim milk with yogurt. Either way, your pressed cheese will be delicious. Always listen to your body! You can drink the remaining whey or use it for making pancakes.

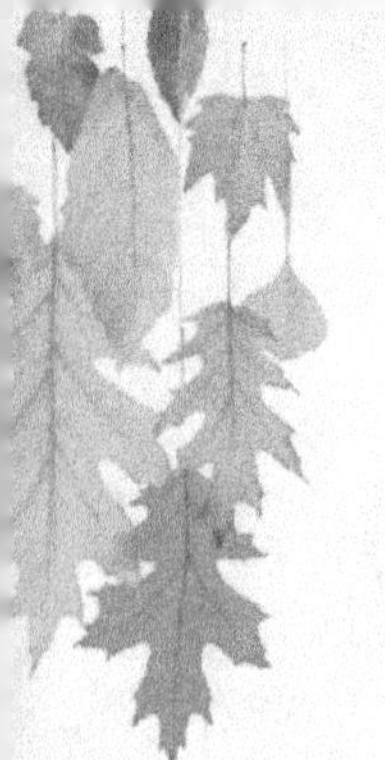

INGREDIENTS

1 liter (~35 fl oz) skim milk *(organic)*
or
1 liter (~35 fl oz) whole milk *(bio)*
1 cup store-bought low-fat (*or* fat-free) yogurt *(bio)*
or
1 cup homemade yogurt
or
200 ml (sweet) cream *(organic)*
1 tablespoon unrefined rock salt
3 eggs *(organic)*

PREPARATION

1. Add salt to milk.
2. Bring milk to a boil.
3. Mix together eggs and cream/yogurt.
4. Add mixture to boiling milk.
5. Stir milk with wooden spoon until well blended.
6. Let milk boil until curds separate from whey.
7. Let curdled milk cool.
8. Leave curdled milk in a strain until no more whey comes out.
9. Serve at room temperature.

You Matter!

1. Take four gorgeous pictures of your culinary result.

2. Write down your impressions of the recipe.

a. Did you like it?

____

b. Was it difficult?

____

c. Did you find all the ingredients?

____

d. Did you make any changes to the recipe to better suit your dietary needs?

____

____

e. Will you cook it again?

____

f. Will you share it with your family and friends?

____

g. How did it make your body feel?

____

____

h. How were you feeling before cooking the recipe?

____

____

i. How were you feeling after eating the culinary result?

____

____

WHEY PANCAKES

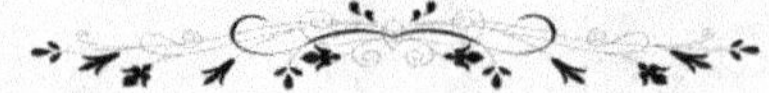

Here is what you can do with the liquid whey from homemade cheese.
This recipe is both healthy and nutritious, not to mention easy to cook.
You can also celebrate your acceptance of anything that you can't control with these tasty pancakes.

Type of Meal	Healthy Snack Breakfast
Type of Dish	Vegetarian Lacto-Ovo-Vegetarian Non-Vegetarian
Preparation Time	Approximately 5 minutes
Cooking Time	Approximately 30 minutes
Servings	8
The AilamA® Cookbook advises You	You can add more flour so that the batter isn't too runny. Or you can choose not to use all the liquid. Instead of coconut milk, you can use coconut water.

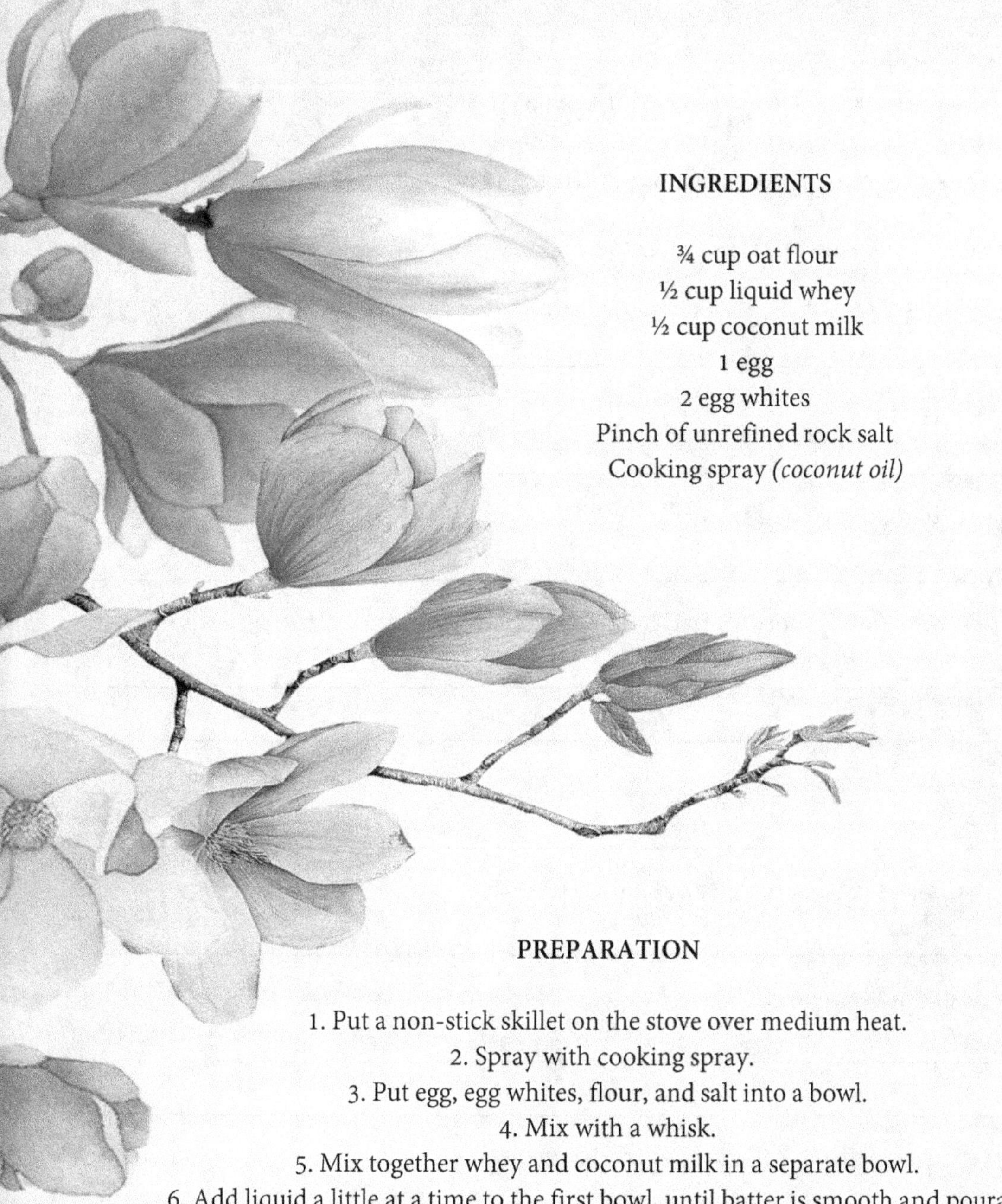

INGREDIENTS

¾ cup oat flour
½ cup liquid whey
½ cup coconut milk
1 egg
2 egg whites
Pinch of unrefined rock salt
Cooking spray *(coconut oil)*

PREPARATION

1. Put a non-stick skillet on the stove over medium heat.
2. Spray with cooking spray.
3. Put egg, egg whites, flour, and salt into a bowl.
4. Mix with a whisk.
5. Mix together whey and coconut milk in a separate bowl.
6. Add liquid a little at a time to the first bowl, until batter is smooth and pourable.
7. Using a ladle, pour batter into skillet three or four times, depending on the size of skillet.
8. Flip pancakes when bubbles form on top.
9. Serve warm, cold, or at room temperature.
10. Serve simple, with fresh fruit, or with fruit preserve on top.

You Matter!

1. Take four gorgeous pictures of your culinary result.

2. Write down your impressions of the recipe.

a. Did you like it?

____

b. Was it difficult?

____

c. Did you find all the ingredients?

____

d. Did you make any changes to the recipe to better suit your dietary needs?

____

____

e. Will you cook it again?

____

f. Will you share it with your family and friends?

____

g. How did it make your body feel?

____

____

h. How were you feeling before cooking the recipe?

____

____

i. How were you feeling after eating the culinary result?

____

____

SMARTLY DRESSED SALAD

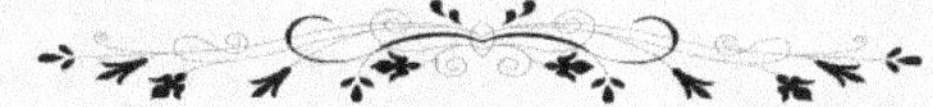

Do you like salads? You most likely do, whether you are a vegetarian or not. Here is a simple recipe with tremendous health benefits.
Allow others to be themselves in order to be allowed to be your true self! This salad can also help you to let go of everything you can't control.

Type of Meal	Breakfast
	Snack
	Lunch
	Supper
Type of Dish	Vegetarian
	Non-Vegetarian
Preparation Time	Approximately 5 minutes
	Approximately 20 minutes, boiling time
	Approximately 10 minutes, baking time
Cooking Time	Approximately 20 minutes
Servings	4
The AilamA® Cookbook advises You	You can dice the onion before putting it in the oven, since it's quite difficult to do it after being baked.

INGREDIENTS

2 handfuls string beans, halved
2 moderate red beets, sliced and quartered
1 medium onion, previously baked, moderately diced
2 tablespoons flaxseed oil, extra virgin, unrefined
½ moderate lemon, juiced *(optional)*
3 tablespoons fresh parsley, washed and chopped
4 gloves garlic, minced
¼ teaspoon unrefined rock salt
¼ teaspoon mixed herbs of your choice *(See also page 6.)*
Chicken breast/beef, minced or cut into bite-sized pieces,
after previously prepared as desired *(non-vegetarian dish)*

PREPARATION

1. Boil beans and beets separately
for more or less than 20 minutes, as desired.
2. Transfer to a mixing bowl.
3. Add oil, garlic, onion, salt, parsley, and spices.
4. Mix well.
5. Add lemon juice for an extra-touch of spiciness. *(optional)*
6. Add chicken breast. *(non-vegetarian dish)*
7. Serve it as a side dish or on its own.

You Matter!

1. Take four gorgeous pictures of your culinary result.

2. Write down your impressions of the recipe.

a. Did you like it?

____

b. Was it difficult?

____

c. Did you find all the ingredients?

____

d. Did you make any changes to the recipe to better suit your dietary needs?

____

____

e. Will you cook it again?

____

f. Will you share it with your family and friends?

____

g. How did it make your body feel?

____

____

h. How were you feeling before cooking the recipe?

____

____

i. How were you feeling after eating the culinary result?

____

____

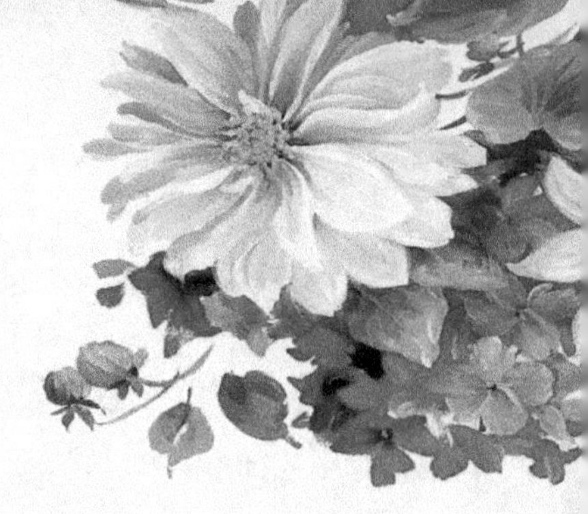

The Recipe of Week 7
MEATY SOUP

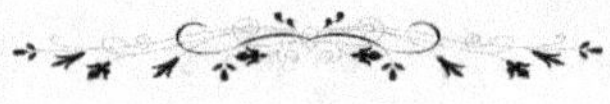

Soups and broths are a great delight in all seasons. Here is a recipe that you'll love. This soup will also support your sincere admiration for someone or something.

Type of Meal	Main Course
	Digestive aid, as the last course of a meal
Type of Dish	Non-Vegetarian
Preparation Time	Approximately 5 minutes
	Approximately 1 hour, soaking time
	Approximately 15 minutes, baking time
Cooking Time	Approximately 45 minutes
Servings	4
The AilamA® Cookbook advises You	Poultry breast can also be slightly broiled before adding it to the soup. That will keep it soft and tender.

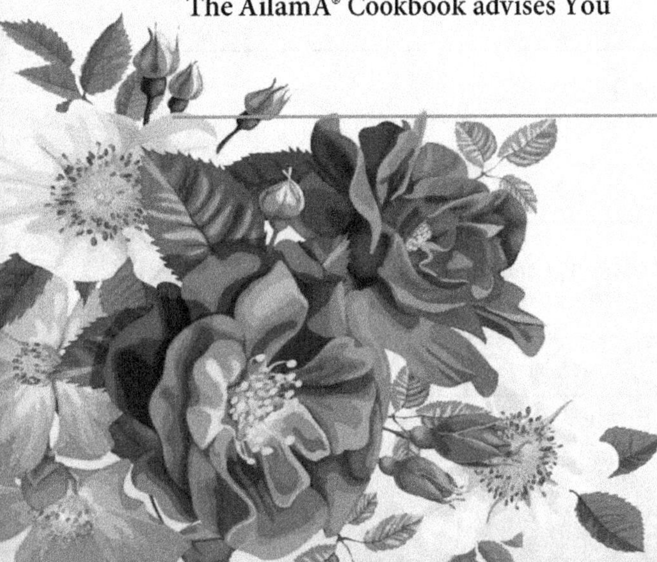

INGREDIENTS

1 handful seaweed, previously soaked in water for 30 minutes, moderately cut
1 handful broccoli florets, washed, halved
1 handful wood ear mushrooms, previously soaked in water for 1 hour
1 cup peas, washed
2 egg whites
chicken/hen/rooster/turkey stock
chicken/hen/rooster/turkey breast, previously baked
2 teaspoons unrefined rock salt
2 teaspoons mixed herbs of your choice *(See also page 6.)*

PREPARATION

1. Put seaweed, broccoli, mushrooms, and peas into a pot.
2. Pour stock over ingredients.
3. Bring to a boil.
4. Cover with lid.
5. Boil over low heat for 30 minutes.
6. Add salt, herbs, and egg whites.
7. Stir gently.
8. Let content cool for 2 minutes.
9. Add chicken/hen/rooster/turkey breast, cooked as desired.
10. Stir one last time.
11. Serve hot, warm, or at room temperature.

You Matter!

1. Take four gorgeous pictures of your culinary result.

2. Write down your impressions of the recipe.

a. Did you like it?

____

b. Was it difficult?

____

c. Did you find all the ingredients?

____

d. Did you make any changes to the recipe to better suit your dietary needs?

____

____

e. Will you cook it again?

____

f. Will you share it with your family and friends?

____

g. How did it make your body feel?

____

____

h. How were you feeling before cooking the recipe?

____

____

i. How were you feeling after eating the culinary result?

____

____

MILLET PUDDING

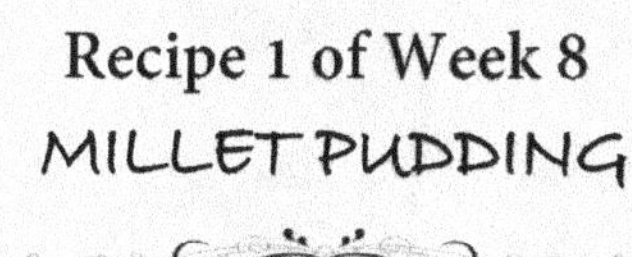
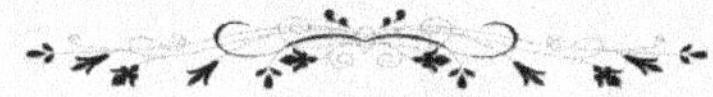

Here is a tasty dish for both meat-eaters and vegetarians. It is packed with healthy nutrients that will boost your energy and will make you feel strong, physically, mentally, and emotionally.
You can also eat it whenever you feel stuck and unmotivated.

Type of Meal	Main Course
	Lunch
Type of dish	Vegetarian
	Ovo-Vegetarian
	Non-Vegetarian
Preparation Time	Approximately 5 minutes
	Approximately 1 hour, soaking time
	Approximately 15 minutes, baking time
	Approximately 15 minutes, boiling time
Cooking Time	Approximately 45 minutes
Servings	4
The AilamA® Cookbook advises You	Rinse millet thoroughly, soak it in spring water for 1 hour, then rinse it again to reduce the amount of starch.

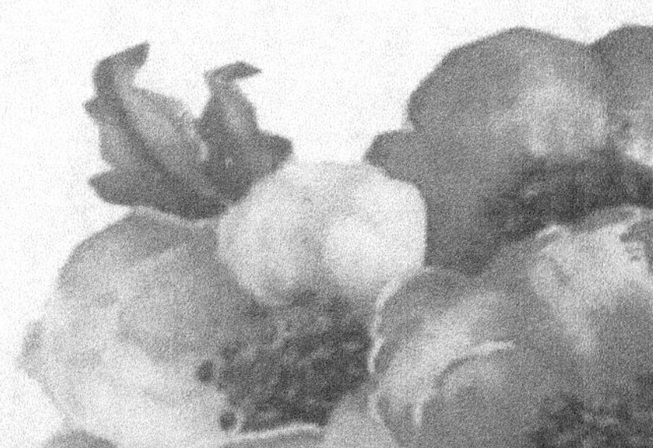

INGREDIENTS

1 organic egg *(optional)*
4 cups millet, previously soaked in water
1 medium onion, previously baked
2 tablespoons extra virgin olive oil
3 cups broccoli florets, previously boiled
2 tablespoons fresh parsley, washed and chopped
¼ teaspoon unrefined sea salt
1½ teaspoons mixed herbs of your choice
(See also page 6.)

PREPARATION

1. Put millet in a pot.
2. Add spring water to cover it.
3. Add 1 teaspoon mixed spice.
4. Bring to a boil.
5. Add water if needed.
6. Let millet simmer for 20 minutes or so, until soft and tender.
(See also pages 61 and 152.)
7. Meanwhile, bake onion and boil broccoli florets.
8. Let millet, onion, and broccoli cool for 5 to 10 minutes.
9. Put boiled millet, oil, egg, salt, onion, parsley, broccoli, and mixed herbs in a blender.
10. Blend until smooth or creamy, as desired.
11. Serve hot, warm, or at room temperature.

You Matter!

1. Take four gorgeous pictures of your culinary result.

2. Write down your impressions of the recipe.

a. Did you like it?

____

b. Was it difficult?

____

c. Did you find all the ingredients?

____

d. Did you make any changes to the recipe to better suit your dietary needs?

____

____

e. Will you cook it again?

____

f. Will you share it with your family and friends?

____

g. How did it make your body feel?

____

____

h. How were you feeling before cooking the recipe?

____

____

i. How were you feeling after eating the culinary result?

____

____

CARO-CREAM

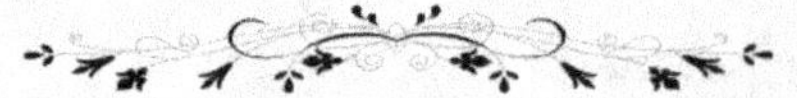

If you are an incurable *chocaholic*, yet you want to stay away from the fat and caffeine content of chocolate, cocoa beans, and cocoa powder, here's a sweet solution to your cocoa-flavored dilemma: the versatile carob cream.

You can also pamper yourself with this tasty dish combined with healthy, fat-free popcorn on cold winter evenings, when binge watching.

Type of Meal	Dessert Snack
Type of Dish	Lacto-Ovo-Vegetarian Non-Vegetarian
Preparation Time	Approximately 1 minute
Cooking Time	0 minutes
Servings	2
The AilamA® Cookbook advises You	You can buy seedless carob pod kibbles, roasted or dried, from any health food store. If you find them dry or fresh and want to roast them at home, keep them in the oven at a low temperature for about 10 minutes so that they won't get burned. (*See also pages 32, 85, and 253.*)

INGREDIENTS

4 tablespoons carob powder, organic
1 small cup warm spring water
¼ teaspoon roasted seeds of your choice *(optional)*
½ teaspoon roasted nuts of your choice *(optional)*
1 large bowl fat-free popcorn, unsalted, prepared at home in ceramic pan *(optional)*

PREPARATION

1. Mix carob powder with water in a glass bowl.
2. Stir until creamy.
3. Add more water or more powder to get a runnier or thicker consistency.
4. Stir until well blended.
5. Add seeds or nuts. *(optional)*
6. Add popcorn. *(optional)*
7. Mix well.
8. Serve it by itself or on homemade bread. *(See also pages 63 and 171.)*

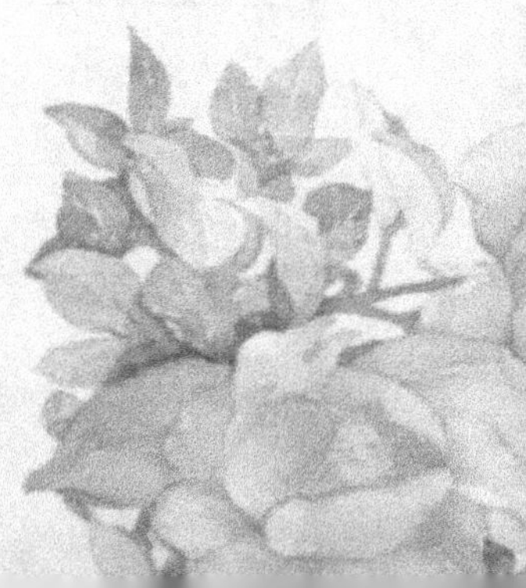

You Matter!

1. Take four gorgeous pictures of your culinary result.

2. Write down your impressions of the recipe.

a. Did you like it?

____

b. Was it difficult?

____

c. Did you find all the ingredients?

____

d. Did you make any changes to the recipe to better suit your dietary needs?

____

____

e. Will you cook it again?

____

f. Will you share it with your family and friends?

____

g. How did it make your body feel?

____

____

h. How were you feeling before cooking the recipe?

____

____

i. How were you feeling after eating the culinary result?

____

____

The Recipe of Week 9
CRANBERRY SALAD

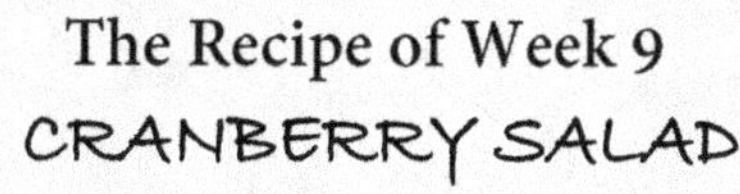

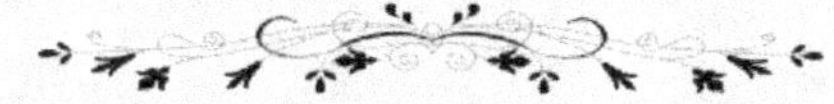

These combinations will make you savor every mouthful of this new salad.
Also, eat this salad whenever something holds you in eager anticipation.

Type of Meal	Breakfast
	Snack
	Lunch
	Supper
Type of Dish	Vegetarian
	Ovo-Vegetarian
	Non-Vegetarian
Preparation Time	Approximately 5 minutes
Cooking Time	Approximately 1 minute
Servings	2
The AilamA® Cookbook advises You	Lettuce can be cut with a wooden knife or can be torn to bits by hand.

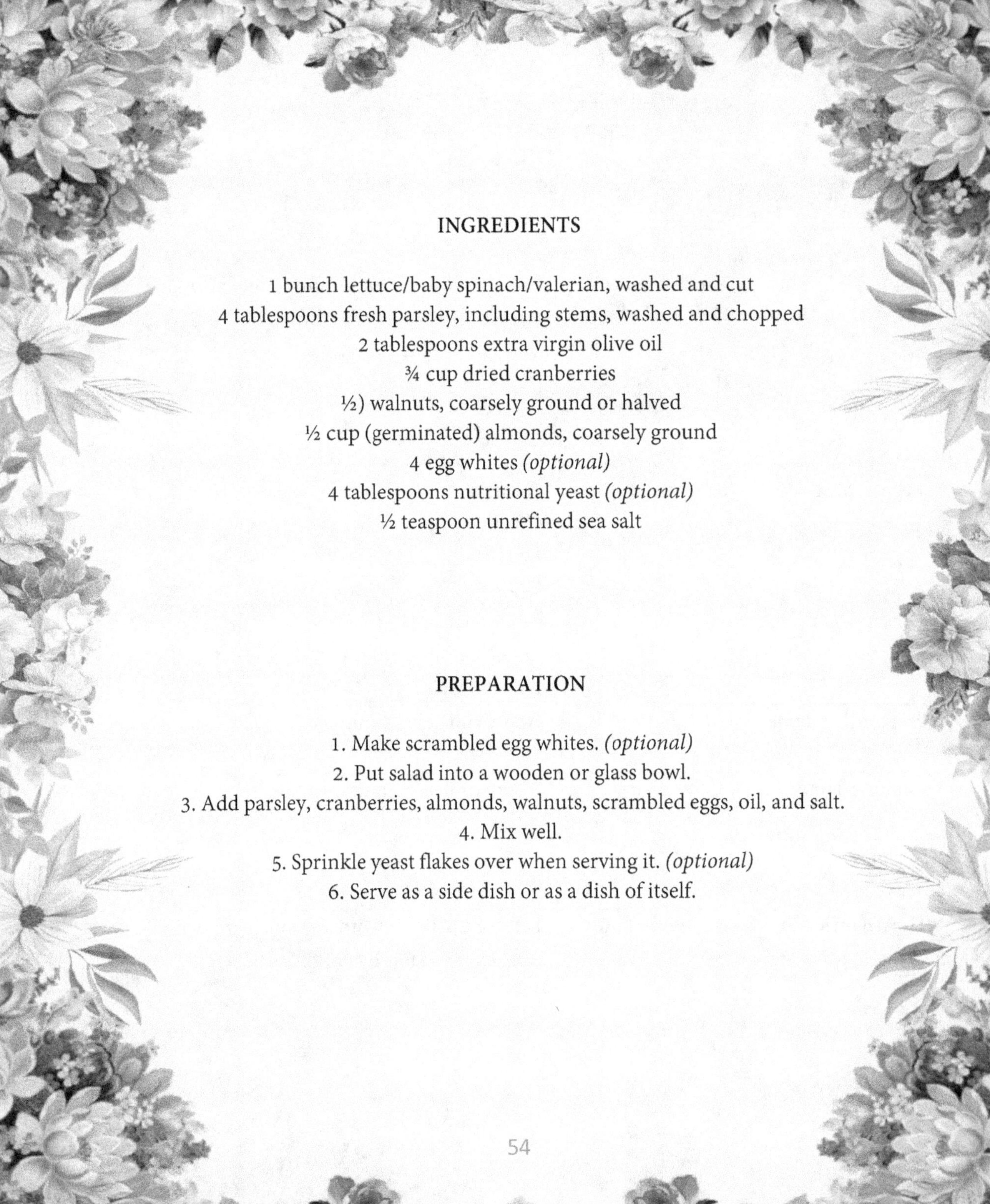

INGREDIENTS

1 bunch lettuce/baby spinach/valerian, washed and cut
4 tablespoons fresh parsley, including stems, washed and chopped
2 tablespoons extra virgin olive oil
¾ cup dried cranberries
½) walnuts, coarsely ground or halved
½ cup (germinated) almonds, coarsely ground
4 egg whites *(optional)*
4 tablespoons nutritional yeast *(optional)*
½ teaspoon unrefined sea salt

PREPARATION

1. Make scrambled egg whites. *(optional)*
2. Put salad into a wooden or glass bowl.
3. Add parsley, cranberries, almonds, walnuts, scrambled eggs, oil, and salt.
4. Mix well.
5. Sprinkle yeast flakes over when serving it. *(optional)*
6. Serve as a side dish or as a dish of itself.

You Matter!

1. Take four gorgeous pictures of your culinary result.

2. Write down your impressions of the recipe.

a. Did you like it?

____

b. Was it difficult?

____

c. Did you find all the ingredients?

____

d. Did you make any changes to the recipe to better suit your dietary needs?

____

____

e. Will you cook it again?

____

f. Will you share it with your family and friends?

____

g. How did it make your body feel?

____

____

h. How were you feeling before cooking the recipe?

____

____

i. How were you feeling after eating the culinary result?

____

____

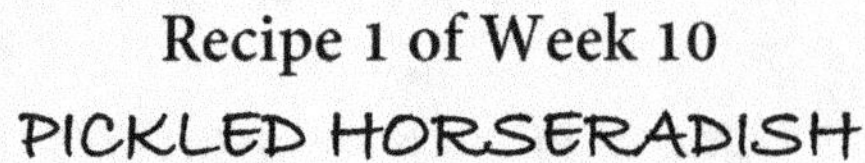

PICKLED HORSERADISH

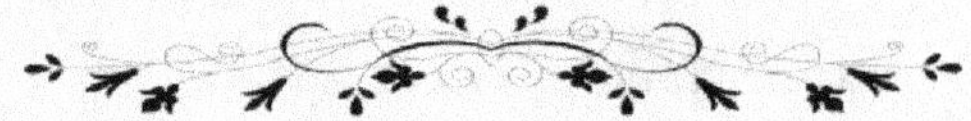

Here is the healthiest way to preserve horseradish.
This strong spice can also give a much-needed boost to your confidence.

Type of Meal	Lunch Supper
Type of Dish	Vegetarian Non-Vegetarian
Preparation Time	Approximately 10 minutes
Cooking Time	0 minutes
Servings	1 small jar
The AilamA® Cookbook advises You	Horseradish is a pungent yet very healthy condiment. You can add it to many dishes, such as sushi, meats, broths, or even salads.

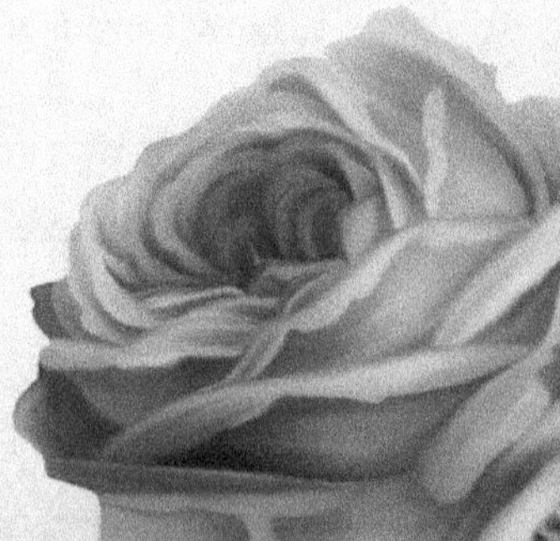

INGREDIENTS

4 medium horseradish roots, grated
3 moderate lemons, juiced
2 teaspoons unrefined rock salt

PREPARATION

1. Grate horseradish small.
2. Put it in a glass jar.
3. Add lemon juice and salt.
4. Mix well.
5. Seal the jar with a perfect-sized lid,
preferably covered by a screw-on ring.
6. Refrigerate.
7. Serve with meats, soups, or sushi.

You Matter!

1. Take four gorgeous pictures of your culinary result.

2. Write down your impressions of the recipe.

a. Did you like it?

____

b. Was it difficult?

____

c. Did you find all the ingredients?

____

d. Did you make any changes to the recipe to better suit your dietary needs?

____

____

e. Will you cook it again?

____

f. Will you share it with your family and friends?

____

g. How did it make your body feel?

____

____

h. How were you feeling before cooking the recipe?

____

____

i. How were you feeling after eating the culinary result?

____

____

BIG SUSHI

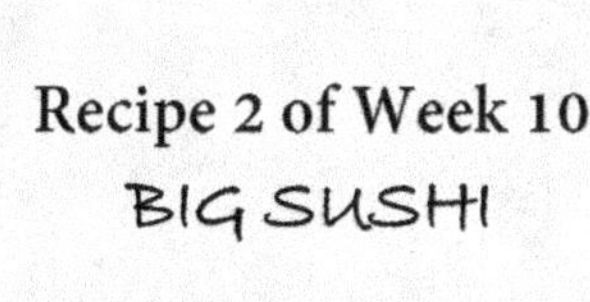

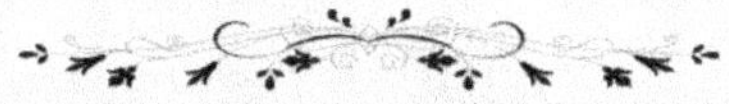

Here is a rapid sushi recipe, using only healthy ingredients. You can also share this dish with an old friend to honor your long friendship.

Type of Meal	Main Course
	Appetizer
	Snack
Type of Dish	Pesco-Ovo-Vegetarian
	Non-Vegetarian
Preparation Time	Approximately 10 minutes
	Approximately 20 minutes, boiling time
	Approximately 1 hour, soaking time *(optional)*
Cooking Time	Approximately 20 minutes
Servings	4
The AilamA® Cookbook advises You	You need to buy a bamboo sushi mat and a pack of nori sheets for this recipe. You can find them in supermarket seafood departments. Nori seaweed is normally sold in thin, dried sheets and is used to wrap sushi. You can help sesame seeds germinate by soaking them in spring water for 1 hour.

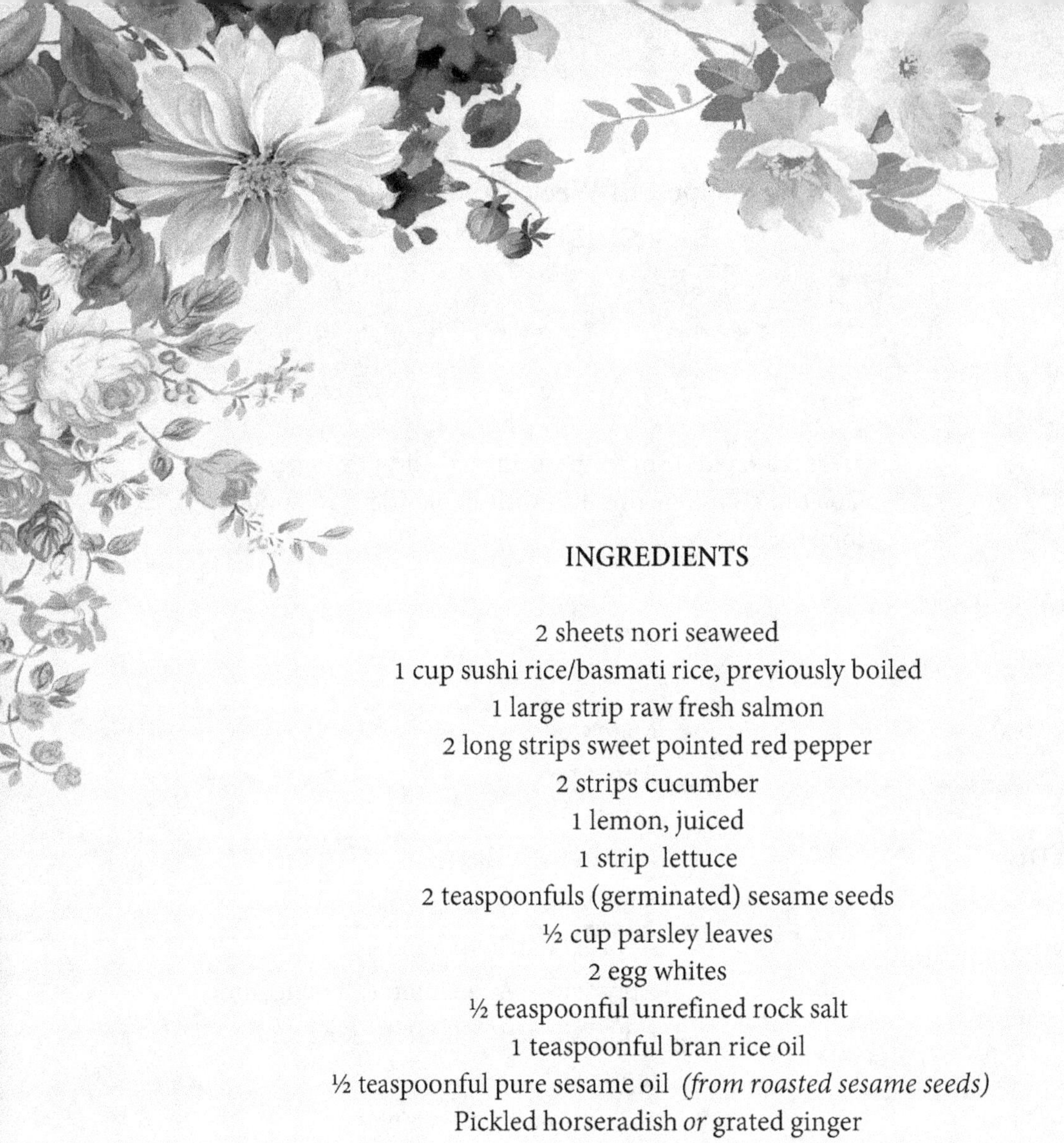

INGREDIENTS

2 sheets nori seaweed
1 cup sushi rice/basmati rice, previously boiled
1 large strip raw fresh salmon
2 long strips sweet pointed red pepper
2 strips cucumber
1 lemon, juiced
1 strip lettuce
2 teaspoonfuls (germinated) sesame seeds
½ cup parsley leaves
2 egg whites
½ teaspoonful unrefined rock salt
1 teaspoonful bran rice oil
½ teaspoonful pure sesame oil *(from roasted sesame seeds)*
Pickled horseradish *or* grated ginger

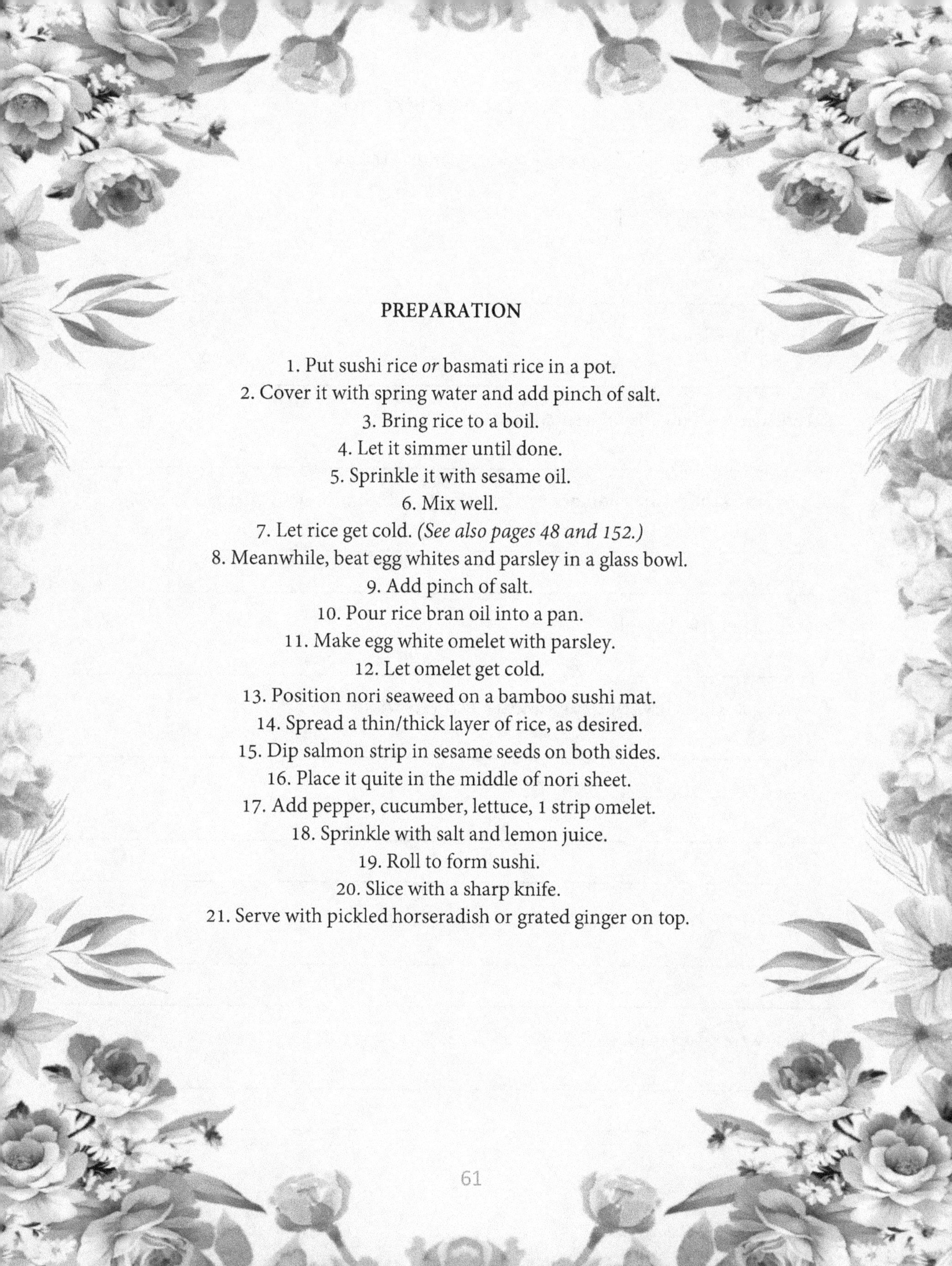

PREPARATION

1. Put sushi rice *or* basmati rice in a pot.
2. Cover it with spring water and add pinch of salt.
3. Bring rice to a boil.
4. Let it simmer until done.
5. Sprinkle it with sesame oil.
6. Mix well.
7. Let rice get cold. *(See also pages 48 and 152.)*
8. Meanwhile, beat egg whites and parsley in a glass bowl.
9. Add pinch of salt.
10. Pour rice bran oil into a pan.
11. Make egg white omelet with parsley.
12. Let omelet get cold.
13. Position nori seaweed on a bamboo sushi mat.
14. Spread a thin/thick layer of rice, as desired.
15. Dip salmon strip in sesame seeds on both sides.
16. Place it quite in the middle of nori sheet.
17. Add pepper, cucumber, lettuce, 1 strip omelet.
18. Sprinkle with salt and lemon juice.
19. Roll to form sushi.
20. Slice with a sharp knife.
21. Serve with pickled horseradish or grated ginger on top.

You Matter!

1. Take four gorgeous pictures of your culinary result.

2. Write down your impressions of the recipe.

a. Did you like it?

____

b. Was it difficult?

____

c. Did you find all the ingredients?

____

d. Did you make any changes to the recipe to better suit your dietary needs?

____

____

e. Will you cook it again?

____

f. Will you share it with your family and friends?

____

g. How did it make your body feel?

____

____

h. How were you feeling before cooking the recipe?

____

____

i. How were you feeling after eating the culinary result?

____

____

BREAD BOOSTER

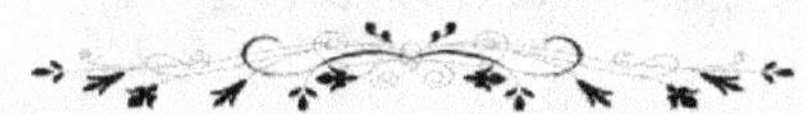

It's important for you to have a bread machine in your house.
Most people eat bread with almost anything.
Why not consuming one that suits your own individuality?
Enjoy your customized bread and be grateful for everything you are and have got !

Type of Meal	Snack Side Dish
Type of Dish	Lacto-Ovo-Vegetarian Non-Vegetarian
Preparation Time	Approximately 5 minutes
Cooking Time	Approximately 4-6 hours
Servings	1 loaf of 700 g (25 oz)
The AilamA® Cookbook advises You	If you use fresh baker's yeast, keep it at room temperature for at least 2 hours before adding it to your bread dough. You can use only one or two types of flour of your choice, if you feel like making the recipe simpler than it is.

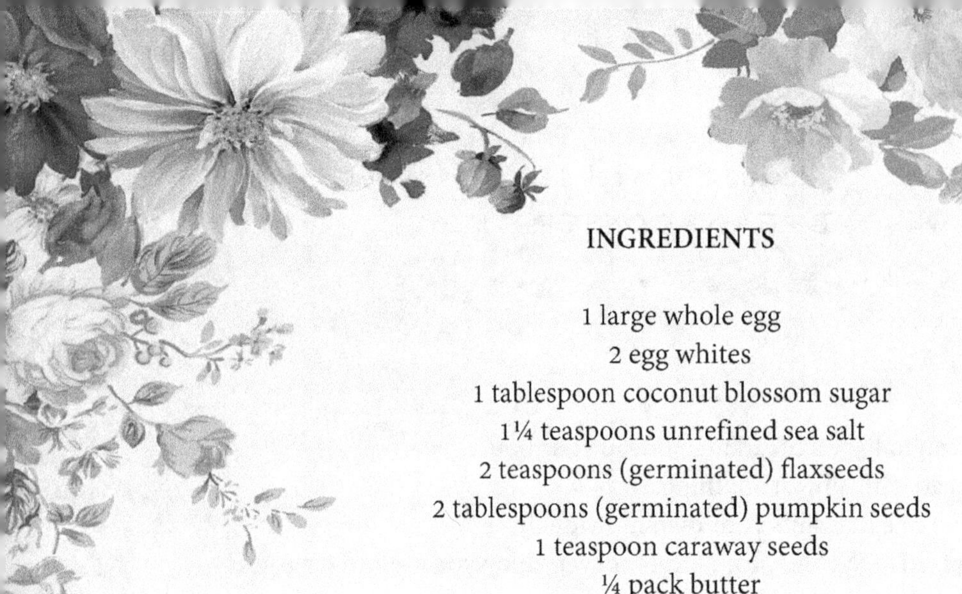

INGREDIENTS

1 large whole egg
2 egg whites
1 tablespoon coconut blossom sugar
1¼ teaspoons unrefined sea salt
2 teaspoons (germinated) flaxseeds
2 tablespoons (germinated) pumpkin seeds
1 teaspoon caraway seeds
¼ pack butter
or
4 tablespoons rice bran oil
350 g (13 oz) rice flour
100 g (3.6 oz) millet flour
50 g (1.8 oz) buckwheat flour
100 g (3.6 oz) quinoa flour
2 tablespoons hemp flour
½ glass spring water *(adjustable quantity)*
½ teaspoon chicory powder *(optional)*
1 teaspoon dried thyme
1 teaspoon dried oregano
1 pack fresh baker's yeast

PREPARATION

1. Put water, agave syrup, salt, flaxseeds, pumpkin seeds, caraway seeds, herbs, thyme, oregano, egg, egg whites, and butter into bread machine's baking pan.
2. Add flour combination, chicory, and yeast.
3. Select **Brown Bread** setting.
4. Bake.
5. Serve with soups, cheese, vegetables, butter, or other spreads.

You Matter!

1. Take four gorgeous pictures of your culinary result.

2. Write down your impressions of the recipe.

a. Did you like it?

____

b. Was it difficult?

____

c. Did you find all the ingredients?

____

d. Did you make any changes to the recipe to better suit your dietary needs?

____

____

e. Will you cook it again?

____

f. Will you share it with your family and friends?

____

g. How did it make your body feel?

____

____

h. How were you feeling before cooking the recipe?

____

____

i. How were you feeling after eating the culinary result?

____

____

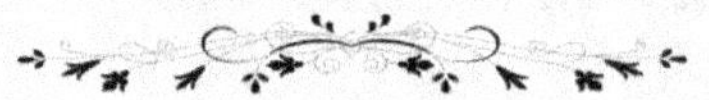

FLUFFY CAKE

Here is the recipe of a sweet dish packed with good protein, and so much more. Also, you can eat this cake whenever you want to feel invincible.

Type of Meal	Snack
	Dessert
Type of Dish	Ovo-Vegetarian
	Non-Vegetarian
Preparation Time	Approximately 10 minutes
Cooking Time	Approximately 1 hour
Servings	16 pieces
The AilamA® Cookbook advises You	Egg yolks are good, but they won't help a sluggish gallbladder at all if they are too many. Egg whites, on the other hand, are light and a safe source of protein for anyone.

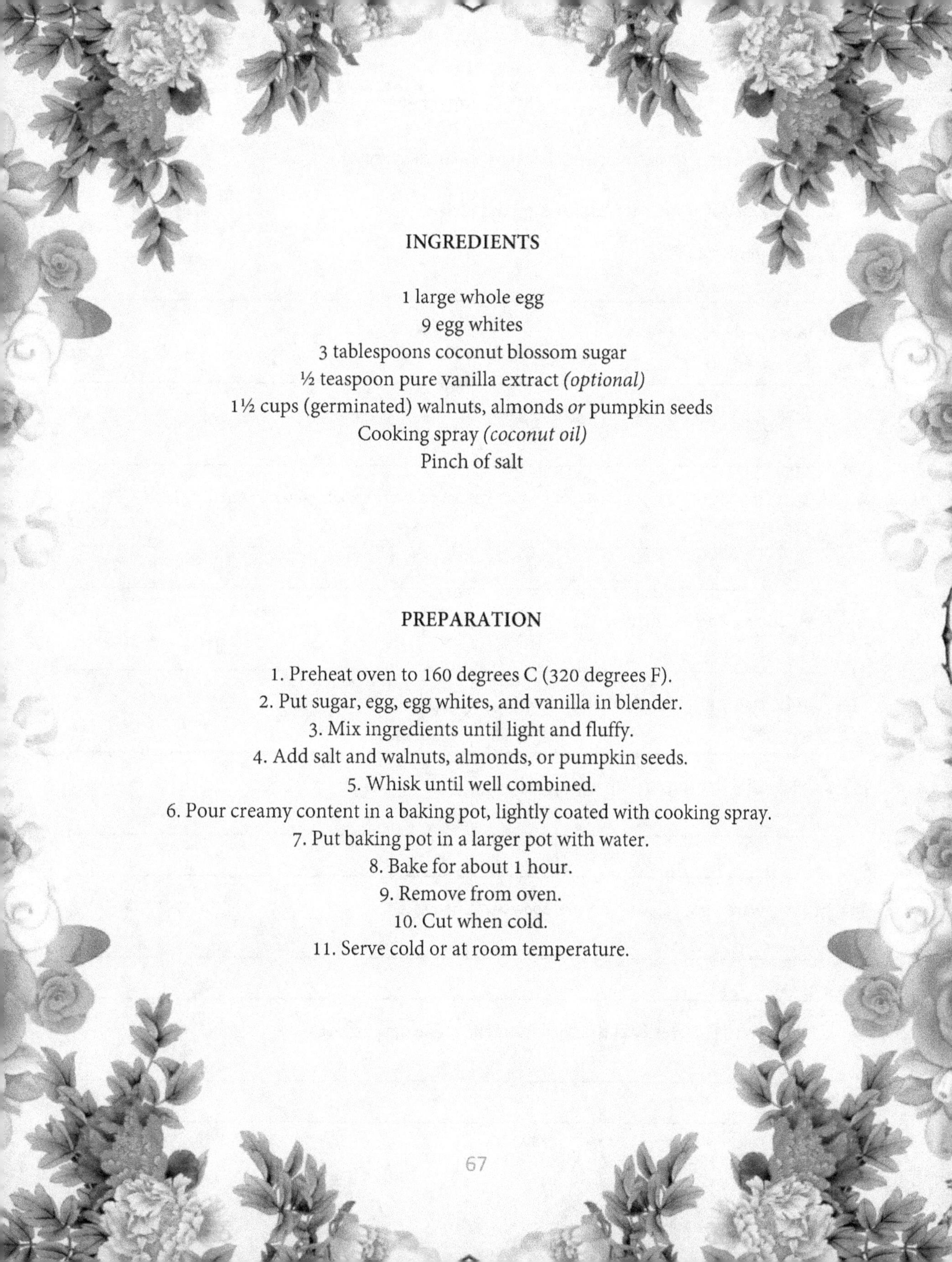

INGREDIENTS

1 large whole egg
9 egg whites
3 tablespoons coconut blossom sugar
½ teaspoon pure vanilla extract *(optional)*
1½ cups (germinated) walnuts, almonds *or* pumpkin seeds
Cooking spray *(coconut oil)*
Pinch of salt

PREPARATION

1. Preheat oven to 160 degrees C (320 degrees F).
2. Put sugar, egg, egg whites, and vanilla in blender.
3. Mix ingredients until light and fluffy.
4. Add salt and walnuts, almonds, or pumpkin seeds.
5. Whisk until well combined.
6. Pour creamy content in a baking pot, lightly coated with cooking spray.
7. Put baking pot in a larger pot with water.
8. Bake for about 1 hour.
9. Remove from oven.
10. Cut when cold.
11. Serve cold or at room temperature.

You Matter!

1. Take four gorgeous pictures of your culinary result.

2. Write down your impressions of the recipe.

a. Did you like it?

____

b. Was it difficult?

____

c. Did you find all the ingredients?

____

d. Did you make any changes to the recipe to better suit your dietary needs?

____

____

e. Will you cook it again?

____

f. Will you share it with your family and friends?

____

g. How did it make your body feel?

____

____

h. How were you feeling before cooking the recipe?

____

____

i. How were you feeling after eating the culinary result?

____

____

CHOCO-NUT

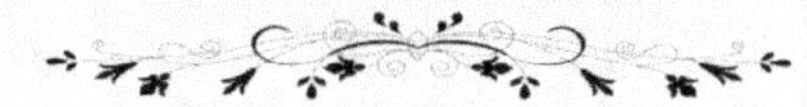

Homemade sweets are healthy dishes when they are prepared with simple, high-quality ingredients.
Here is a nutritious snack for both rainy and shiny days.
It can also be a trustworthy companion whenever you have to pull an all-nighter to further study or work.

Type of Meal	Dessert
	Snack
Type of Dish	Lacto-Ovo-Vegetarian
	Non-Vegetarian
Time of Preparing	Approximately 1 minute
Cooking Time	Approximately 8 minutes
Servings	6
The AilamA® Cookbook advises You	Healthy sweets are great snacks but poor desserts. When eaten alone, or even before main meals, they help combat fatigue, providing you with a boost of energy and nutrients for the whole day.

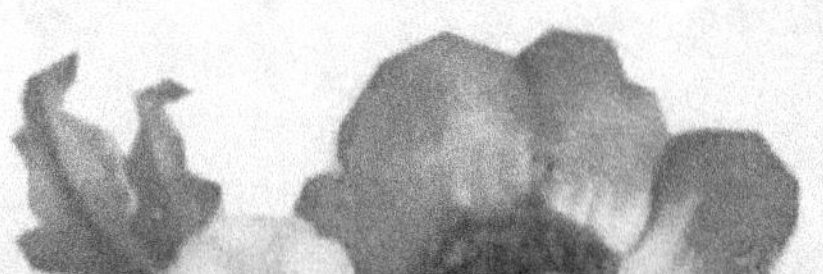

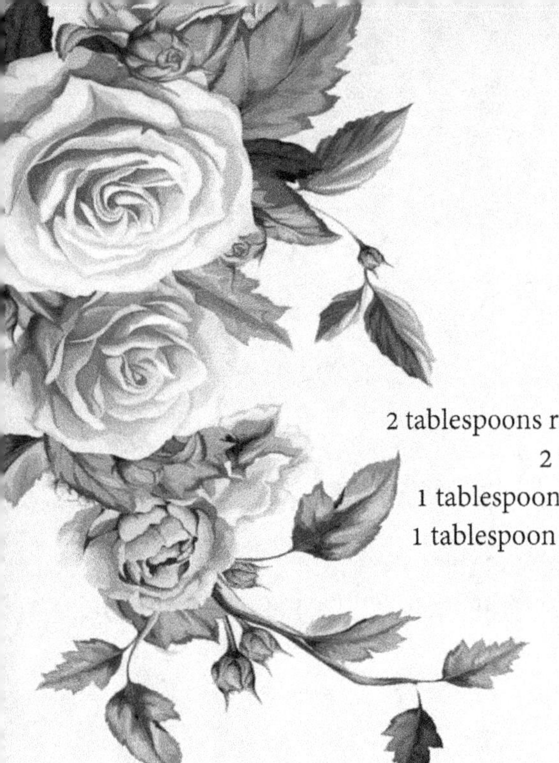

INGREDIENTS

1 egg
2 teaspoons raw honey *or* agave syrup
or
10 drops stevia extract
2 tablespoons raw milk butter *or* ghee *(clarified butter)* or cocoa butter
2 teaspoons cocoa powder *or* carob powder
1 tablespoon (germinated) walnuts, coarsely chopped or blended
1 tablespoon (germinated) almonds, coarsely chopped or blended
Spring water *(optional)*

PREPARATION

1. Mix egg with sweetener in a pot.
2. Stir until blended.
3. Put pot in a bain-marie (double boiler).
4. Add butter.
5. Stir until well blended and creamy.
6. Add cocoa or carob powder, walnuts, and almonds.
7. Mix well for 1 minute or so.
8. Add spring water if too thick. *(optional)*
9. Remove pot from heat.
10. Let it cool for 2 minutes.
11. Pour content in small ceramic *or* glass pots.
12. Serve warm, cold, chilled, or frozen.

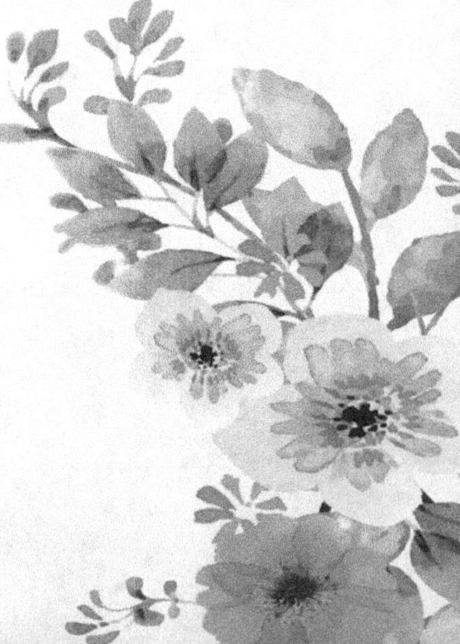

You Matter!

1. Take four gorgeous pictures of your culinary result.

2. Write down your impressions of the recipe.

a. Did you like it?

____

b. Was it difficult?

____

c. Did you find all the ingredients?

____

d. Did you make any changes to the recipe to better suit your dietary needs?

____

____

e. Will you cook it again?

____

f. Will you share it with your family and friends?

____

g. How did it make your body feel?

____

____

h. How were you feeling before cooking the recipe?

____

____

i. How were you feeling after eating the culinary result?

____

____

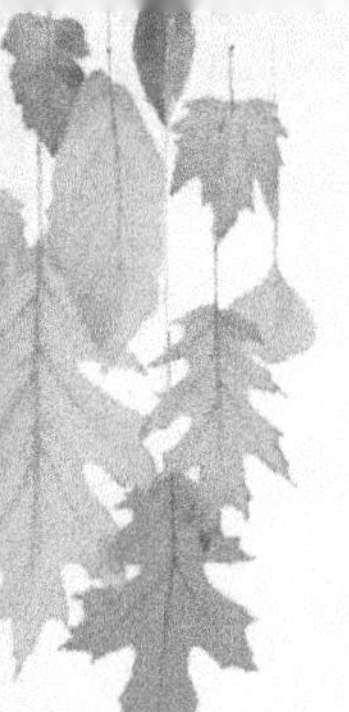

HOMEMADE YOGURT

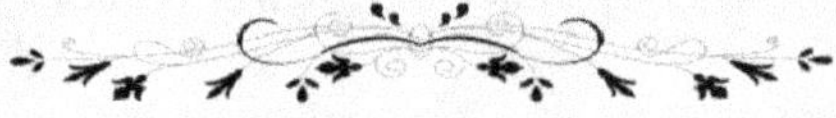

Here is the easiest recipe ever for yogurt.

If you are diabetic or if you suffer from poor digestion due to thyroid, liver, adrenal, and/or gallbladder dysfunctions, use the recipe below exactly as it is.

If you are perfectly healthy, you can opt for organic whole milk. It's also up to you how much fat your whole milk will contain. Just listen to your body!

You can also have this healthy dairy product whenever you feel you have reached a plateau in your romantic life.

Type of Meal	Snack Main Course
Type of Dish	Lacto-Vegetarian Non-Vegetarian
Preparation Time	Approximately 60 minutes
Cooking Time	Approximately 4 hours
Servings	10
The AilamA® Cookbook advises You	After making your first batch, you'll use your own yogurt as a starter. The longer the yogurt sits in the oven (over the established time frame), the thicker it becomes.

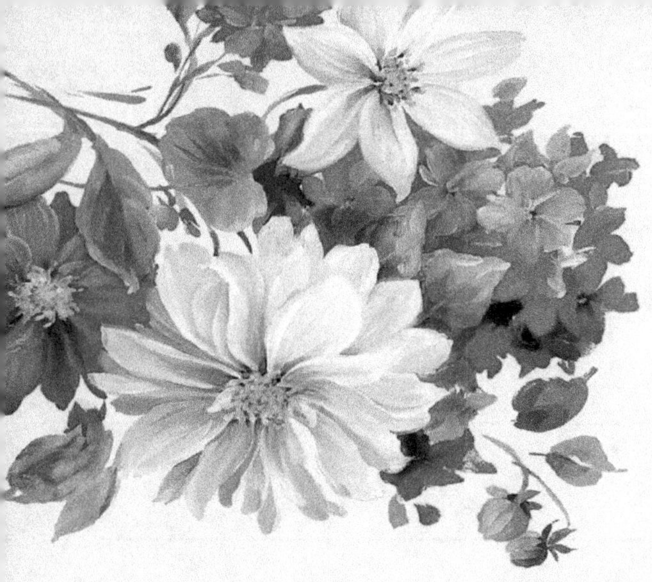

INGREDIENTS

1 liter (~35 fl oz) skim milk *(bio)*
1 cup store-bought low-fat *or* fat-free yogurt *(bio)*, with active cultures in it

PREPARATION

1. Bring milk to a boil.
2. Let milk simmer for 5 minutes.
3. Let milk cool until warm to the touch.
4. Dissolve yogurt in a cup of warm milk.
5. Pour thinned yogurt into warm milk.
6. Stir milk with wooden spoon until well mixed.
7. Place pot in turned-off oven.
8. Turn on oven light.
or
Wrap pot in towel.
9. Let yogurt sit for 4 hours or more.
10. Keep yogurt in the refrigerator.
11. Serve with bread, fruit, cereals, or by itself.

You Matter!

1. Take four gorgeous pictures of your culinary result.

2. Write down your impressions of the recipe.

a. Did you like it?

____

b. Was it difficult?

____

c. Did you find all the ingredients?

____

d. Did you make any changes to the recipe to better suit your dietary needs?

____

____

e. Will you cook it again?

____

f. Will you share it with your family and friends?

____

g. How did it make your body feel?

____

____

h. How were you feeling before cooking the recipe?

____

____

i. How were you feeling after eating the culinary result?

____

____

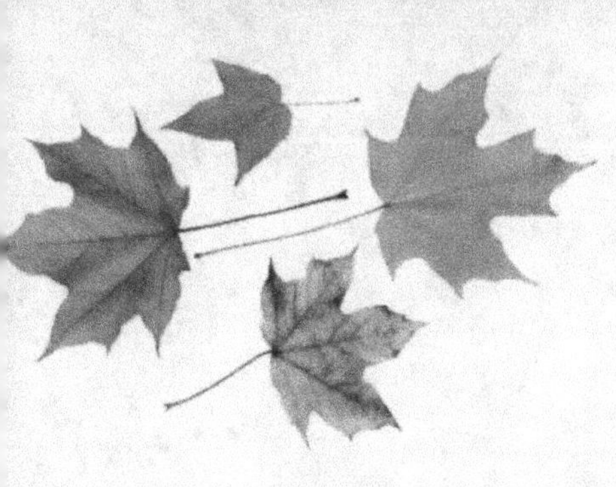
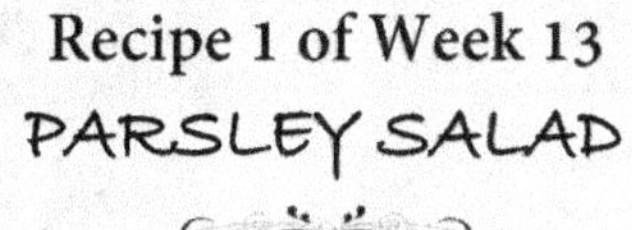
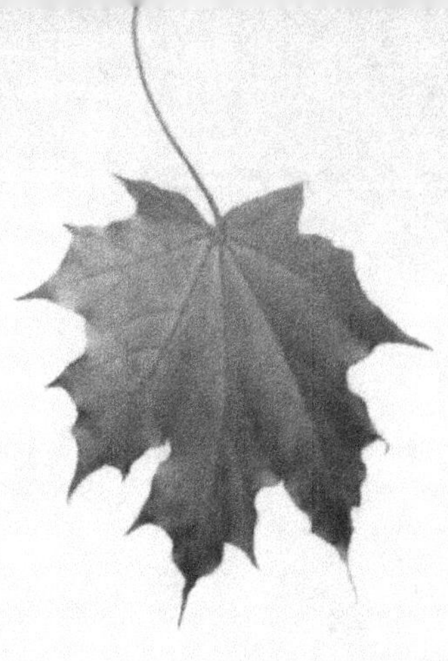

PARSLEY SALAD

Here is yet another deceivingly simple recipe with tremendous health benefits. You can also eat this salad to get courage in the face of fear.

Type of Meal	Salad Side Dish
Type of Dish	Vegetarian Non-Vegetarian
Preparation Time	Approximately 5 minutes Approximately 20 minutes, boiling time
Cooking Time	Approximately 20 minutes
Servings	4
The AilamA® Cookbook advises You	Parsley salads taste better the next day, if kept in a lidded glass bowl in the refrigerator. You can replace parsley with arugula or baby spinach if you want.

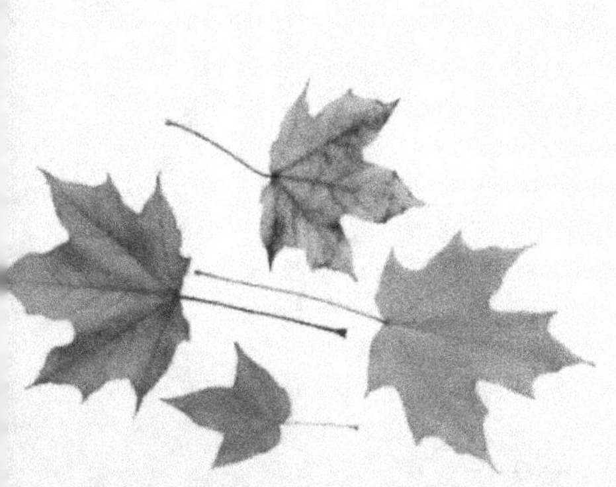
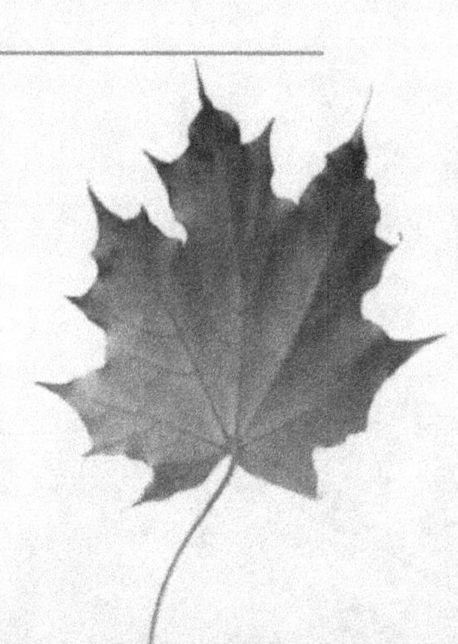

INGREDIENTS

2 moderate red beets, diced small
3 bunches fresh parsley, including stems, washed and chopped
4 tablespoons extra virgin olive oil
½ cup cedar nuts
½ cup (germinated) walnuts, coarsely ground or halved
½ moderate lemon, juiced *(optional)*
½ teaspoon unrefined rock salt

PREPARATION

1. Boil beets for 20 minutes.
2. Transfer to a mixing bowl.
3. Add parsley, oil, salt, cedar nuts, and walnuts.
4. Mix well.
5. Add lemon juice for a sweet-sour taste. *(optional)*
6. Serve with meats or on its own.

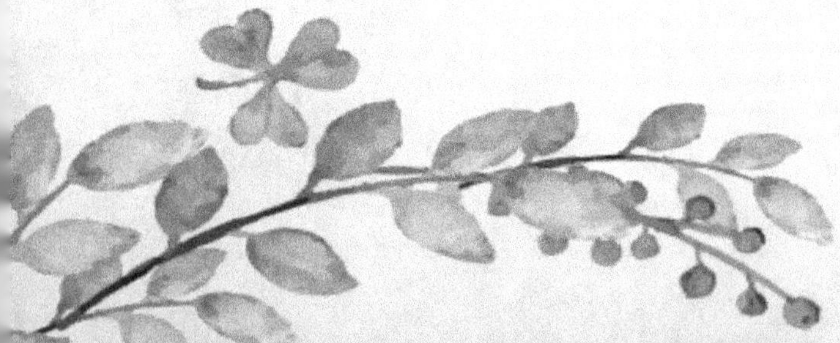

You Matter!

1. Take four gorgeous pictures of your culinary result.

2. Write down your impressions of the recipe.

a. Did you like it?

____

b. Was it difficult?

____

c. Did you find all the ingredients?

____

d. Did you make any changes to the recipe to better suit your dietary needs?

____

____

e. Will you cook it again?

____

f. Will you share it with your family and friends?

____

g. How did it make your body feel?

____

____

h. How were you feeling before cooking the recipe?

____

____

i. How were you feeling after eating the culinary result?

____

____

FIG TRUFFLES

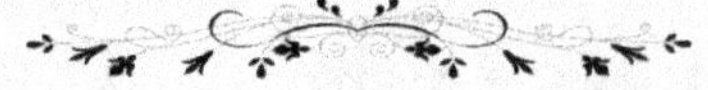

Here is a deceivingly simple recipe for healthy chocolates with natural sugar and lots of dietary fiber.

This sweet dish can also calm you down when you feel overexcited or when you feel insecure about your ability to do something.

Type of Meal	Snack Dessert
Type of Dish	Vegetarian Raw Vegan Non-Vegetarian
Preparation Time	Approximately 5 minutes
Cooking Time	0 minutes
Servings	3
The AilamA® Cookbook advises You	You can use the same recipe to make Date, Prune, Mulberry, or Coconut (Meat) Truffles.

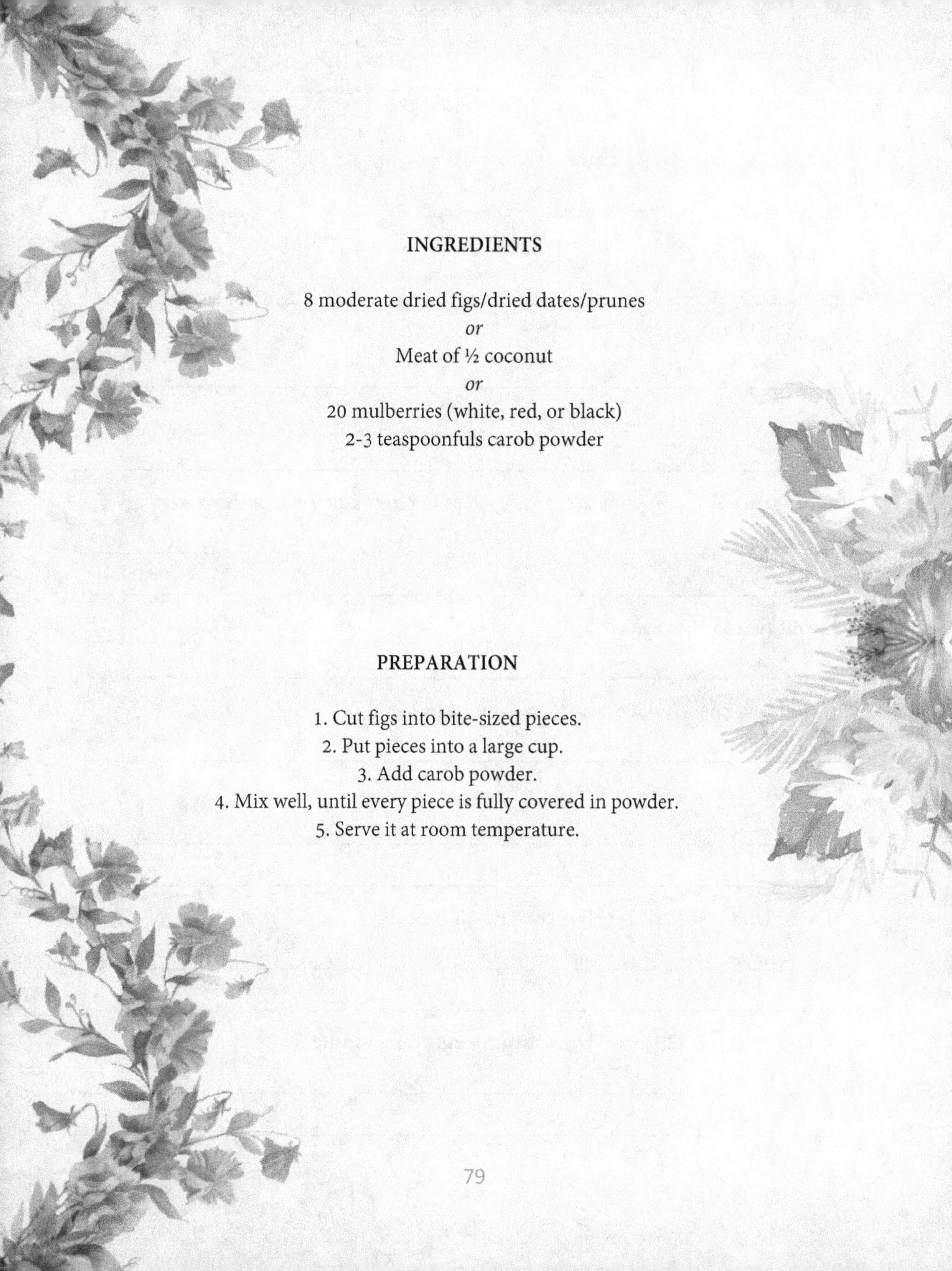

INGREDIENTS

8 moderate dried figs/dried dates/prunes
or
Meat of ½ coconut
or
20 mulberries (white, red, or black)
2-3 teaspoonfuls carob powder

PREPARATION

1. Cut figs into bite-sized pieces.
2. Put pieces into a large cup.
3. Add carob powder.
4. Mix well, until every piece is fully covered in powder.
5. Serve it at room temperature.

You Matter!

1. Take four gorgeous pictures of your culinary result.

2. Write down your impressions of the recipe.

a. Did you like it?

____

b. Was it difficult?

____

c. Did you find all the ingredients?

____

d. Did you make any changes to the recipe to better suit your dietary needs?

____

____

e. Will you cook it again?

____

f. Will you share it with your family and friends?

____

g. How did it make your body feel?

____

____

h. How were you feeling before cooking the recipe?

____

____

i. How were you feeling after eating the culinary result?

____

____

PATTIES

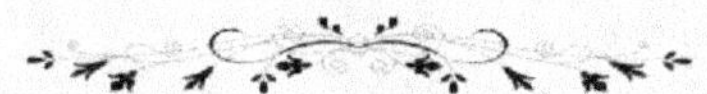

Are you secretly in love with sweets?
Here is a cookie recipe using only healthy ingredients to nourish you and
your family.
Patties could also help you not to overreact to criticism.

Type of Meal	Snack
	Dessert
Type of Dish	Lacto-Ovo-Vegetarian
	Non-Vegetarian
Preparation Time	Approximately 10 minutes
	Approximately 30 minutes, refrigeration time
Cooking Time	Approximately 20 minutes
Servings	16 pieces
The AilamA® Cookbook advises You	Rice, millet, quinoa, and buckwheat are gluten-free grains. You can use their flour as a healthy base for cookies, white sauces, and homemade breads, especially if you are gluten-intolerant.

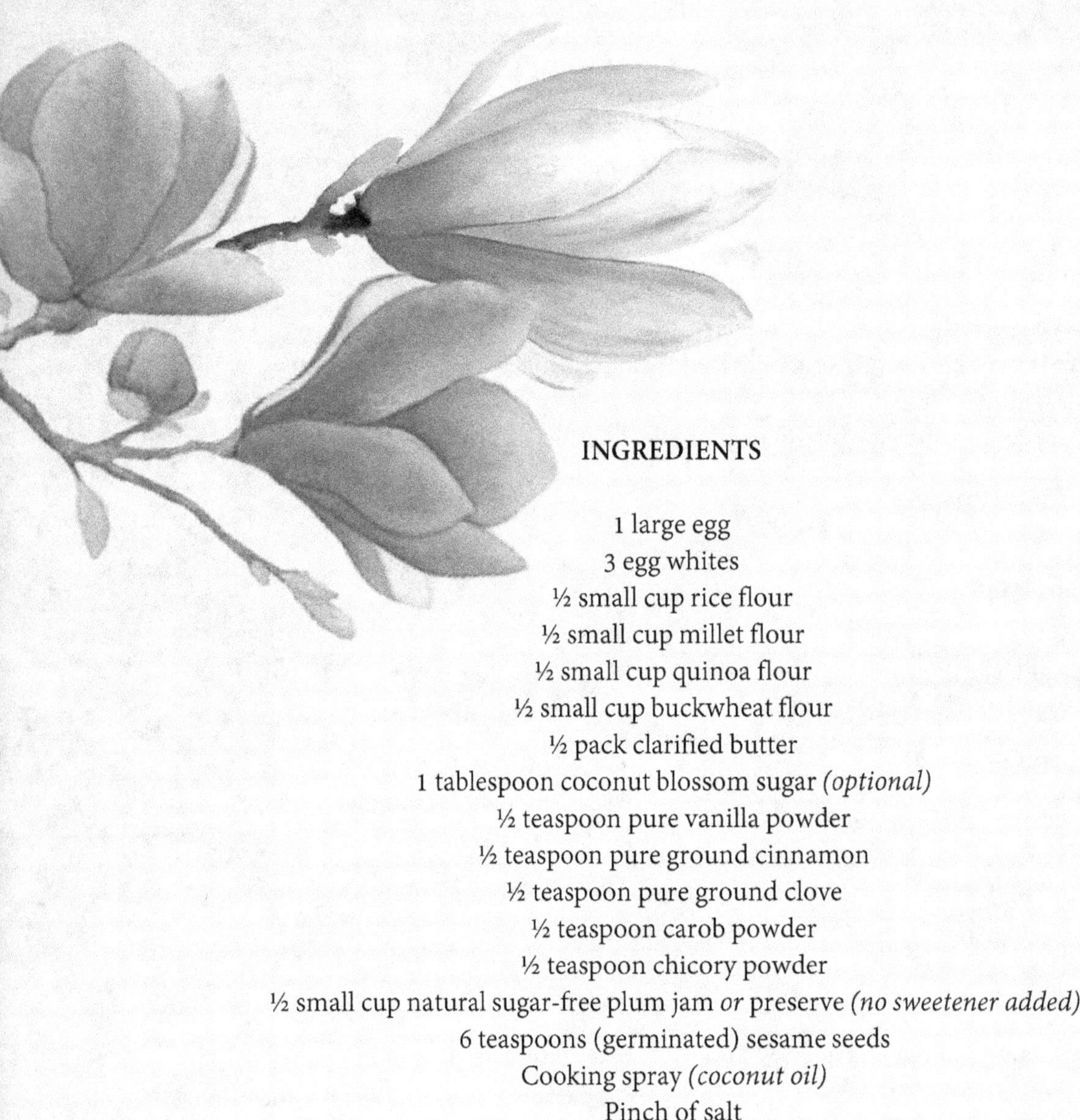

INGREDIENTS

1 large egg
3 egg whites
½ small cup rice flour
½ small cup millet flour
½ small cup quinoa flour
½ small cup buckwheat flour
½ pack clarified butter
1 tablespoon coconut blossom sugar *(optional)*
½ teaspoon pure vanilla powder
½ teaspoon pure ground cinnamon
½ teaspoon pure ground clove
½ teaspoon carob powder
½ teaspoon chicory powder
½ small cup natural sugar-free plum jam *or* preserve *(no sweetener added)*
6 teaspoons (germinated) sesame seeds
Cooking spray *(coconut oil)*
Pinch of salt

PREPARATION

1. Preheat oven to 160 degrees C (320 degrees F).
2. Put butter, sugar, egg, vanilla, clove, cinnamon in a blender.
3. Mix until light and fluffy.
4. Beat egg whites until stiff.
5. Combine butter mixture with egg whites.
6. Blend gently.
7. Add flour, carob and chicory powder, salt, and 4 teaspoons sesame seeds.
8. Whisk until well combined.
9. Add more flour, if needed. *(optional)*
10. Refrigerate batter for 30 minutes.
11. Shape dough into small patties.
12. Place on a baking tray, lightly coated with cooking spray.
13. Add ¼ teaspoon plum jam on each patty.
14. Sprinkle on top with 2 teaspoons sesame seeds.
15. Bake for about 20 minutes or until golden brown.
16. Remove from oven.
17. Serve at room temperature.

You Matter!

1. Take four gorgeous pictures of your culinary result.

2. Write down your impressions of the recipe.

a. Did you like it?

____

b. Was it difficult?

____

c. Did you find all the ingredients?

____

d. Did you make any changes to the recipe to better suit your dietary needs?

____

____

e. Will you cook it again?

____

f. Will you share it with your family and friends?

____

g. How did it make your body feel?

____

____

h. How were you feeling before cooking the recipe?

____

____

i. How were you feeling after eating the culinary result?

____

____

MILK THISTLE CRUNCH

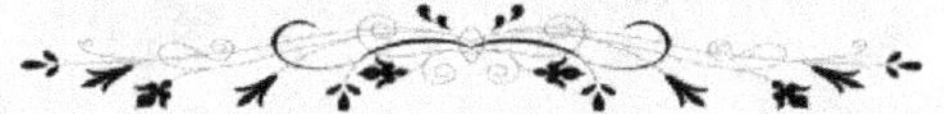

The seeds and leaves of the milk thistle plant are known as powerful liver supporters and detoxifiers, among their many other benefits. The seeds can be eaten completely raw, but they can also be roasted and ground into a caffeine-free, liver-friendly powder. This healthy type of coffee can also give you great comfort in unhappy situations or it can seal your joy whenever you have experienced something good.

Type of Meal	Beverage
Type of Dish	Vegetarian Non-Vegetarian
Preparation Time	Approximately 10 minutes, washing time Approximately 8 hours, soaking time
Cooking Time	Approximately 30 minutes
Servings	10
The AilamA® Cookbook advises You	From time to time, you can replace this magic drink with homemade chicory-root or dandelion-root coffee. Your liver will thank you for whatever option you choose.

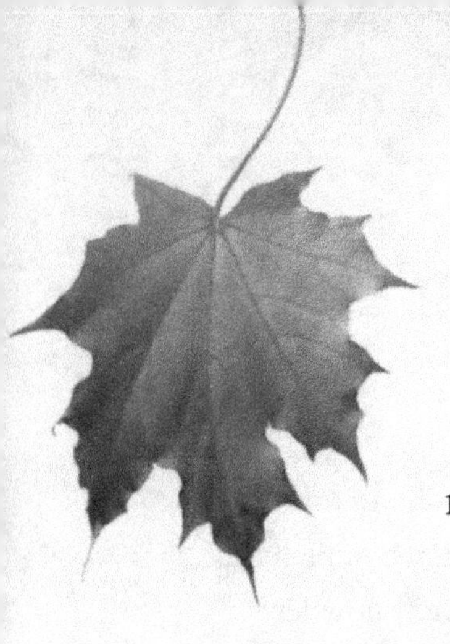
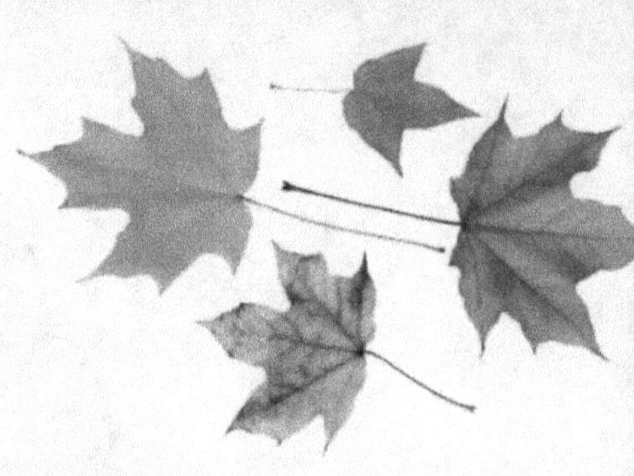

INGREDIENTS

1 cup (or more) milk thistle seeds *(bio, from health food store)*

PREPARATION

1. Wash seeds thoroughly until water comes out clear.
2. Soak seeds in spring water overnight.
3. For optimal results, keep soaked seeds in the refrigerator.
4. Rinse seeds several times.
5. Roast seeds in oven at the lowest temperature setting.
6. Stir seeds occasionally, until they become dark brown (not burned).
7. Let seeds cool.
8. Eat seeds whole, 1 teaspoonful 2-3 times a day.

COFFEE

1. Grind seeds into powder.
2. Bring 1¼ cups spring water to a boil.
3. Add 1 teaspoon milk thistle coffee.
4. Simmer for 5 minutes.
5. Drink it warm or cold.
6. Drink it black.
7. Drink it with coconut water and coconut milk or with the juice from baked apples.
(See also pages 32 and 253.)

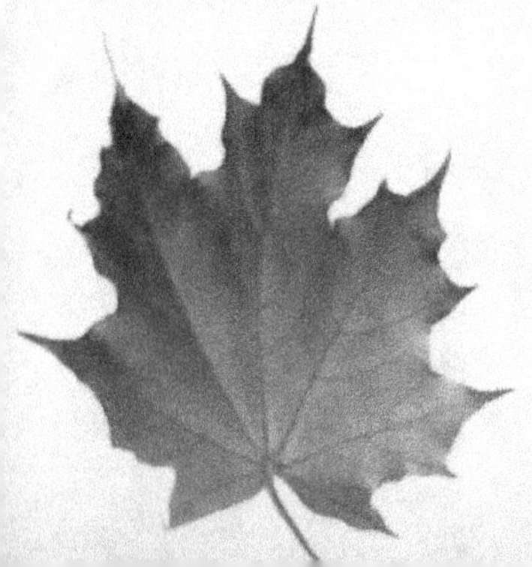
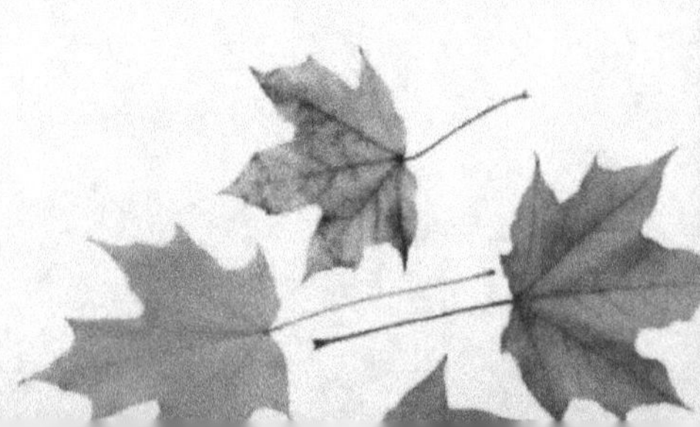

You Matter!

1. Take four gorgeous pictures of your culinary result.

2. Write down your impressions of the recipe.

a. Did you like it?

____

b. Was it difficult?

____

c. Did you find all the ingredients?

____

d. Did you make any changes to the recipe to better suit your dietary needs?

____

____

e. Will you cook it again?

____

f. Will you share it with your family and friends?

____

g. How did it make your body feel?

____

____

h. How were you feeling before cooking the recipe?

____

____

i. How were you feeling after eating the culinary result?

____

____

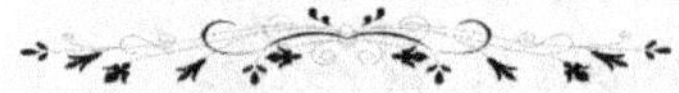

Your mind will set itself free from all sweet-related rigors and interdictions as soon as you have tried this cake recipe.

It can also help you harness love's amazing force.

Type of Meal	Snack
	Dessert
Type of Dish	Lacto-Ovo-Vegetarian
	Non-Vegetarian
Preparation Time	Approximately 10 minutes
Cooking Time	Approximately 1 hour
Servings	6 pieces
The AilamA® Cookbook advises You	You can change the degree of sweetness by adding more or less of the proposed sweetener. You can just taste the cream and decide how sweet it should be.

INGREDIENTS

CAKE BASE

12 egg whites
¼ small cup agave syrup *or* raw honey
or
20 drops stevia extract
or
2 tablespoons coconut blossom sugar
2 cups (germinated) walnuts, almonds, and pumpkin seeds
Cooking spray *(coconut oil)*
Pinch of salt

CHOCOLATE CREAM

1 egg
2 teaspoons agave syrup/raw honey
or
10 drops stevia extract
or
1 tablespoon coconut blossom sugar
2½ teaspoons cocoa powder *or* carob powder
¼ pack cocoa butter *or* clarified butter
Spring water *(optional)*

PREPARATION

CAKE BASE

1. Preheat oven to 160 degrees C (320 degrees F).
2. Put sweetener and egg whites in a blender.
3. Mix until stiff.
4. Add walnuts, almonds, pumpkin seeds, and salt.
5. Whisk gently until well combined.
6. Pour creamy content in a medium or large baking pot, lightly coated with cooking spray.
7. Put baking pot in a larger pot with water.
8. Bake in a bain-marie for about 1 hour.
9. Remove from oven.

CHOCOLATE CREAM

1. Mix egg with sweetener in a pot.
2. Stir until blended.
3. Place a bowl on top of a pot of simmering water on low heat to make a bain-marie (double boiler).
4. Add butter.
5. Stir until well blended and creamy.
6. Add cocoa or carob powder.
7. Mix well for 1 minute or so.
8. Add spring water if too thick. *(optional)*
9. Let cream cool for 5 minutes.
10. Spread it all over the cake base in a thin or thick layer, as preferred.
11. Cut when cold.
12. Serve chilled or at room temperature.

You Matter!

1. Take four gorgeous pictures of your culinary result.

2. Write down your impressions of the recipe.

a. Did you like it?

____

b. Was it difficult?

____

c. Did you find all the ingredients?

____

d. Did you make any changes to the recipe to better suit your dietary needs?

____

____

e. Will you cook it again?

____

f. Will you share it with your family and friends?

____

g. How did it make your body feel?

____

____

h. How were you feeling before cooking the recipe?

____

____

i. How were you feeling after eating the culinary result?

____

____

VEG-SUSHI

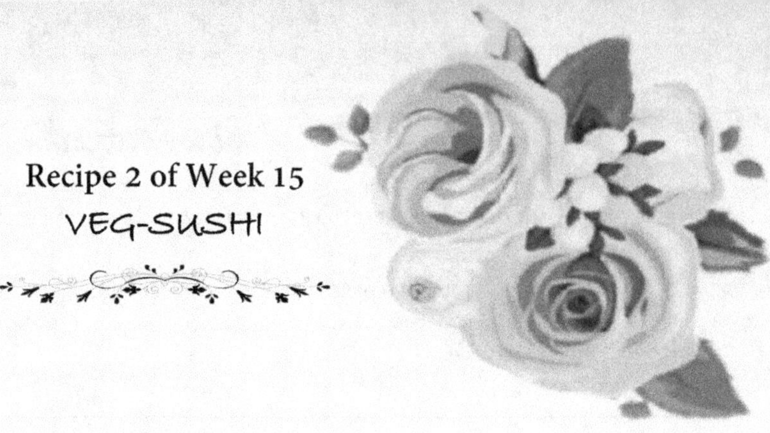

Anything is possible both in your life and in your kitchen if you let your imagination fly above and beyond.

Besides your culinary project 365, you can prepare this special sushi when you are longing to see your ex again.

Type of Meal	Main Course
	Appetizer
	Snack
Type of Dish	Ovo-Vegetarian
Preparation Time	Approximately 10 minutes
	Approximately 20 minutes, boiling time
Cooking Time	Approximately 20 minutes
Servings	4
The AilamA® Cookbook advises You	Omelet doesn't stick very well to the seaweed sheet, so you can wet the nori sheet a little bit before adding the omelet.

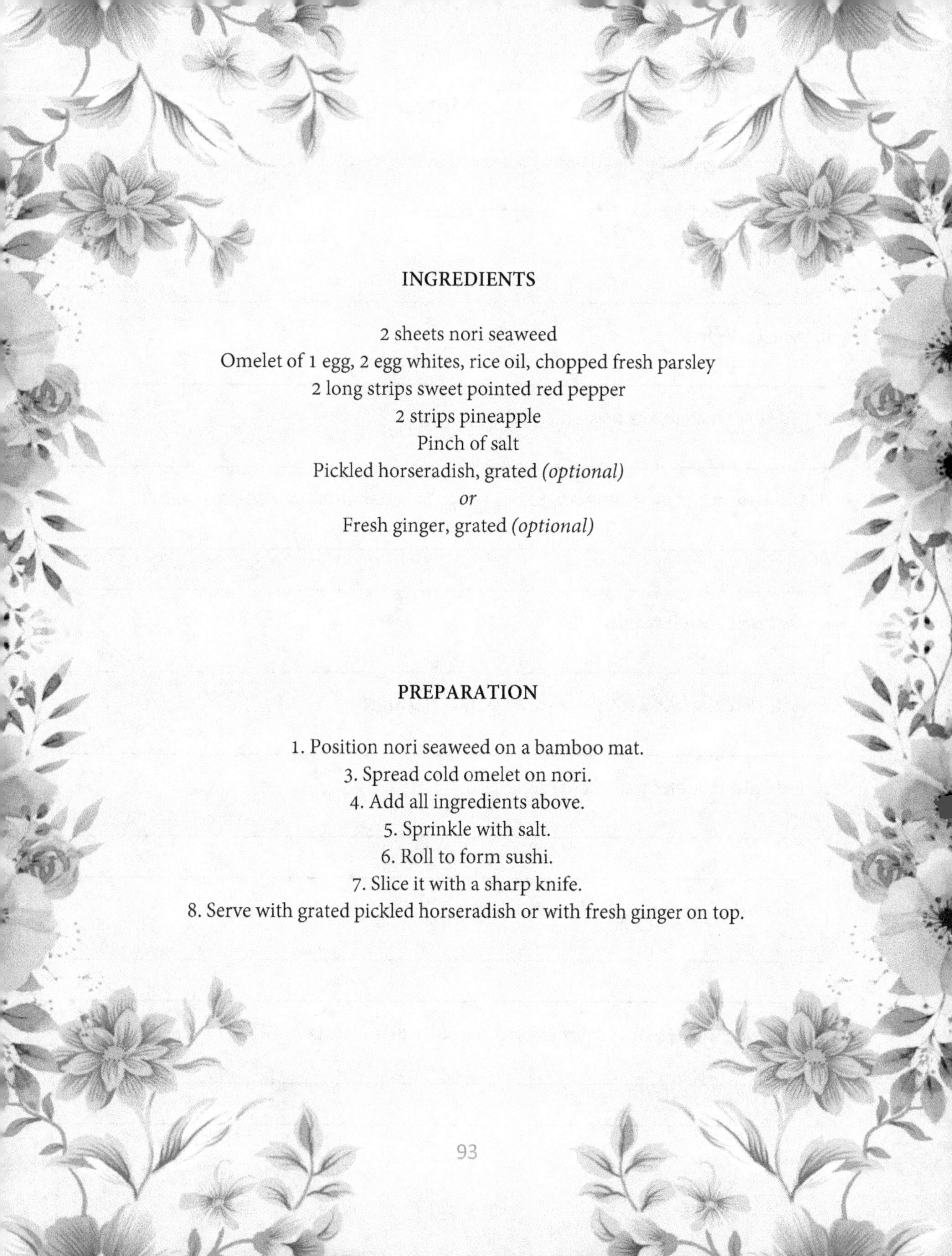

INGREDIENTS

2 sheets nori seaweed
Omelet of 1 egg, 2 egg whites, rice oil, chopped fresh parsley
2 long strips sweet pointed red pepper
2 strips pineapple
Pinch of salt
Pickled horseradish, grated *(optional)*
or
Fresh ginger, grated *(optional)*

PREPARATION

1. Position nori seaweed on a bamboo mat.
3. Spread cold omelet on nori.
4. Add all ingredients above.
5. Sprinkle with salt.
6. Roll to form sushi.
7. Slice it with a sharp knife.
8. Serve with grated pickled horseradish or with fresh ginger on top.

You Matter!

1. Take four gorgeous pictures of your culinary result.

2. Write down your impressions of the recipe.

a. Did you like it?

____

b. Was it difficult?

____

c. Did you find all the ingredients?

____

d. Did you make any changes to the recipe to better suit your dietary needs?

____

____

e. Will you cook it again?

____

f. Will you share it with your family and friends?

____

g. How did it make your body feel?

____

____

h. How were you feeling before cooking the recipe?

____

____

i. How were you feeling after eating the culinary result?

____

____

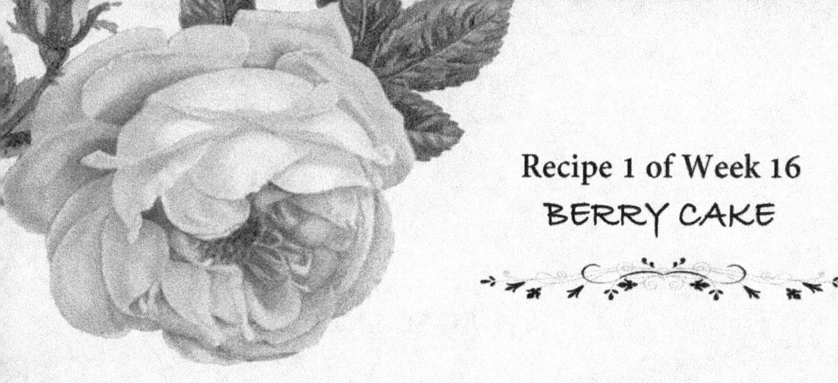

BERRY CAKE

Once you have tried this recipe, it's easy to create your own healthy filling, using whatever fruit you like.

This cake is also about motivating you to be creative in all life circumstances.

Type of Meal	Snack
	Dessert
Type of Dish	Ovo-Vegetarian
	Non-Vegetarian
Preparation Time	Approximately 10 minutes
Cooking Time	Approximately 1 hour
Servings	16 pieces
The AilamA® Cookbook advises You	To see if a cake is done, insert a toothpick in it and see if it comes out clean.

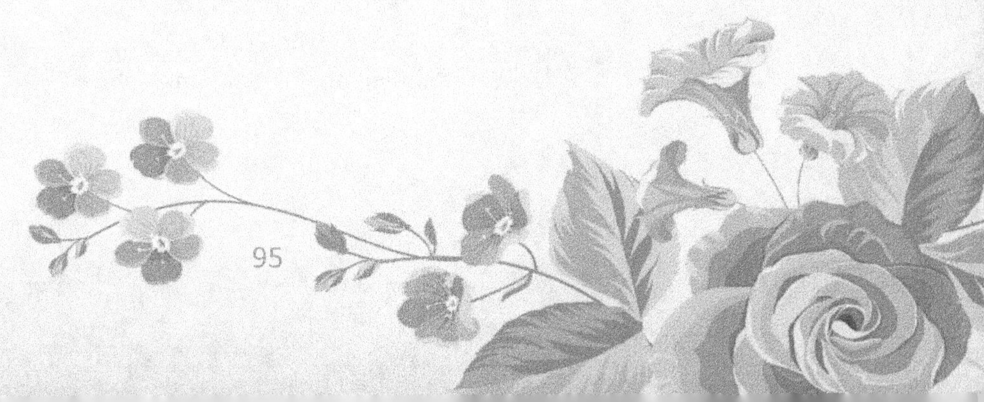

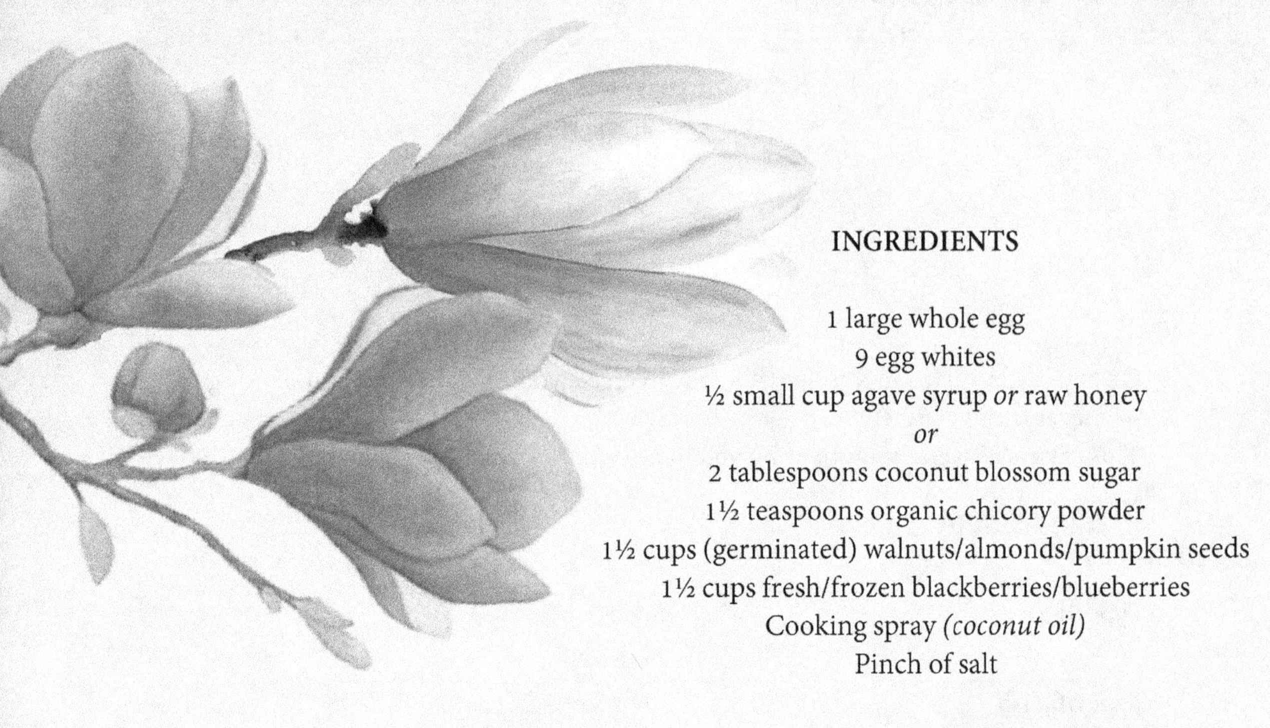

INGREDIENTS

1 large whole egg
9 egg whites
½ small cup agave syrup *or* raw honey
or
2 tablespoons coconut blossom sugar
1½ teaspoons organic chicory powder
1½ cups (germinated) walnuts/almonds/pumpkin seeds
1½ cups fresh/frozen blackberries/blueberries
Cooking spray *(coconut oil)*
Pinch of salt

PREPARATION

1. Preheat oven to 160 degrees C (320 degrees F).
2. Put sweetener and whole egg in a blender.
3. Mix ingredients until light and fluffy.
4. Add walnuts/almonds/pumpkin seeds and salt.
5. Whisk gently until well combined.
6. Beat egg whites until stiff.
7. Mix all ingredients.
8. Pour creamy content in a medium or large baking pot, lightly coated with cooking spray.
9. Add pieces of fruit, lightly pressing them into cream.
10. Put baking pot in a larger pot, filled with water.
11. Bake in a bain-marie for about 1 hour.
12. Remove from oven.
13. Cut when cold.
14. Serve chilled or at room temperature.

You Matter!

1. Take four gorgeous pictures of your culinary result.

2. Write down your impressions of the recipe.

a. Did you like it?

____

b. Was it difficult?

____

c. Did you find all the ingredients?

____

d. Did you make any changes to the recipe to better suit your dietary needs?

____

____

e. Will you cook it again?

____

f. Will you share it with your family and friends?

____

g. How did it make your body feel?

____

____

h. How were you feeling before cooking the recipe?

____

____

i. How were you feeling after eating the culinary result?

____

____

COCKTAIL SKEWERS

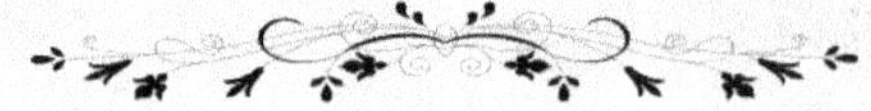

Here is a delicious way of combining meat with vegetables. Skewers can be tasty reminders of the fact that people come together to have fun.

They can thus be a perfect treat for unexpected guests, since they take so little time to prepare.

Type of Meal	Main Course Lunch Supper
Type of Dish	Vegetarian Non-Vegetarian
Preparation Time	Approximately 10 minutes
Cooking Time	Approximately 6 minutes
Servings	6 skewers
The AilamA® Cookbook advises You	Instead of meat, you can add as many vegetables as you can on the wooden sticks, if you are a vegetarian.

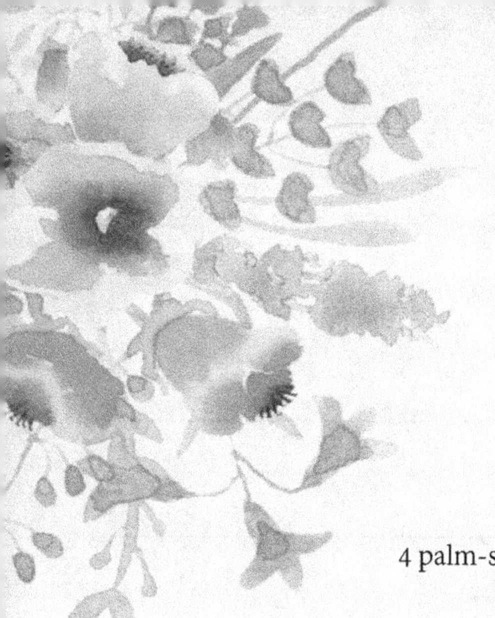

INGREDIENTS

2 zucchini, moderately sliced
3 sweet pointed red peppers, halved
3 onions, cut into moderate chunks
½ lemon, juiced *(optional)*
4 palm-sized pieces of meat (beef, veal, chicken breast, etc.),
cut into moderate chunks
3 moderate fillets of cod/salmon/trout
½ teaspoon unrefined rock salt
½ teaspoon mixed herbs of your choice *(See also page 6.)*

PREPARATION

1. Skewer all ingredients on 6 wooden sticks, alternating meat with vegetables.
2. Use all types of meat (if you have more than one) and all types of vegetables on each skewer.
3. Sprinkle them with salt, lemon juice, and seasonings.
4. Broil them for approximately 6 minutes.
5. Serve hot, warm, or at room temperature.

You Matter!

1. Take four gorgeous pictures of your culinary result.

2. Write down your impressions of the recipe.

a. Did you like it?

____

b. Was it difficult?

____

c. Did you find all the ingredients?

____

d. Did you make any changes to the recipe to better suit your dietary needs?

____

____

e. Will you cook it again?

____

f. Will you share it with your family and friends?

____

g. How did it make your body feel?

____

____

h. How were you feeling before cooking the recipe?

____

____

i. How were you feeling after eating the culinary result?

____

____

HOMEMADE PÂTÉ

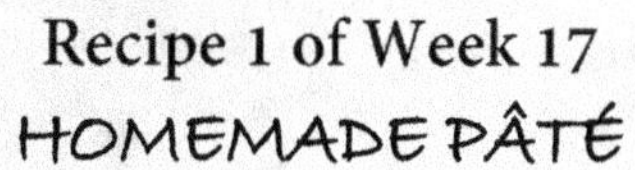

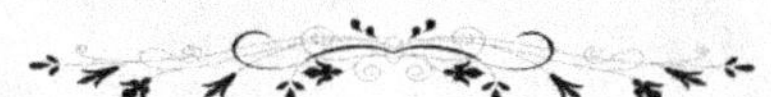

Here is a tasty, nutrient-dense dish for meat-eaters. This pâté can also be your comfort food when you are visited by bittersweet memories.

Type of Meal	Main Course
	Snack
Type of Dish	Non-Vegetarian
Preparation Time	Approximately 5 minutes
	Approximately 10 minutes, boiling time
	Approximately 10 minutes, baking time
Cooking Time	Approximately 10 minutes
Servings	4
The AilamA® Cookbook advises You	When the other ingredients are hot, raw eggs become a natural smoother and taste enhancer.

INGREDIENTS

1 egg
2 large beef liver chunks, largely cut
1 medium onion, baked
1 cup extra virgin olive oil
¼ teaspoon unrefined sea salt
½ moderate lemon, juiced *(optional)*
1½ teaspoons mixed herbs of your choice *(See also page 6.)*

PREPARATION

1. Put liver chunks in a pot.
2. Add spring water to cover them.
3. Boil them for 10 minutes with 1 teaspoon mixed herbs.
4. Bake onion for 10 minutes.
5. Put boiled liver, oil, salt, egg, onion, and ½ mixed herbs in a blender.
6. Blend until smooth.
7. Add lemon juice until desired taste is obtained. *(optional)*
8. Transfer to a mixing bowl.
9. Whisk it until smooth as desired.
10. Serve at room temperature, on slices of sweet red pepper or homemade bread.

You Matter!

1. Take four gorgeous pictures of your culinary result.

2. Write down your impressions of the recipe.

a. Did you like it?

____

b. Was it difficult?

____

c. Did you find all the ingredients?

____

d. Did you make any changes to the recipe to better suit your dietary needs?

____

____

e. Will you cook it again?

____

f. Will you share it with your family and friends?

____

g. How did it make your body feel?

____

____

h. How were you feeling before cooking the recipe?

____

____

i. How were you feeling after eating the culinary result?

____

____

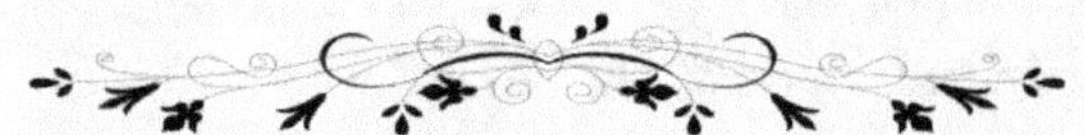

BUTTER FRUIT COCKTAIL

Do you like fruit?
Here is a healthy way to cook them for better digestion.
Also, eat this tasty combination when you feel ashamed of yourself for making a great fuss about something quite insignificant.

Type of Meal	Side Dish
	Dessert
	Breakfast
	Snack
Type of Dish	Lacto-Vegetarian
	Non-Vegetarian
Preparation Time	Approximately 2 minutes
Cooking Time	Approximately 1 minute
Servings	4
The AilamA® Cookbook advises You	Frying pans are excellent for healthy cooking (not frying!), since they are generally made of cast iron, which is a perfect heat conductor as well as a safe cookware material.

INGREDIENTS

2 large ripe bananas, moderately sliced on the diagonal
2 medium pineapple slices, cut into moderate chunks
½ red grapefruit, cut into moderate chunks
1 medium mango fruit, cut into moderate chunks
2 tablespoons cocoa butter *or* coconut butter
¼ teaspoon ground cinnamon
¼ teaspoon ground clove
2 tablespoons (germinated) sesame seeds

PREPARATION

1. Melt butter in a heavy pan over low heat.
2. Add banana chunks.
3. Gently stir for at least 30 seconds.
4. Add pineapple, mango, grapefruit, and sesame seeds.
5. Stir gently for at least 30 seconds.
6. Remove pan from heat.
7. Transfer sautéed fruit into glass bowls.
8. Sprinkle with cinnamon and clove.
9. Serve hot.

You Matter!

1. Take four gorgeous pictures of your culinary result.

2. Write down your impressions of the recipe.

a. Did you like it?

____

b. Was it difficult?

____

c. Did you find all the ingredients?

____

d. Did you make any changes to the recipe to better suit your dietary needs?

____

____

e. Will you cook it again?

____

f. Will you share it with your family and friends?

____

g. How did it make your body feel?

____

____

h. How were you feeling before cooking the recipe?

____

____

i. How were you feeling after eating the culinary result?

____

____

SWEET-SOUR CHICKEN

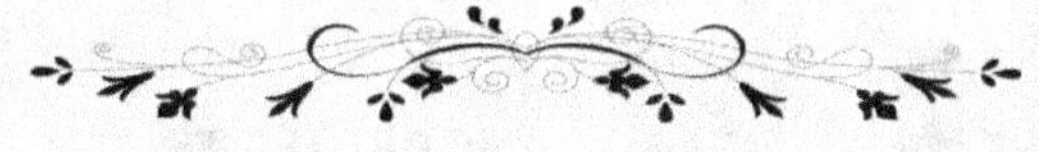

Here is yet another tasty, nutrient-dense dish for meat-eaters.
You can also eat it to ignore the thoughts telling you that you've been rather a disappointment to your family and friends.

Type of Meal	Main Course Lunch Dinner
Type of Dish	Non-Vegetarian
Preparation Time	Approximately 10 minutes
Cooking Time	Approximately 5 minutes
Servings	4
The AilamA® Cookbook advises You	Any kind of meat will do in this recipe (turkey, beef, pork, venison), but chicken is probably the best.

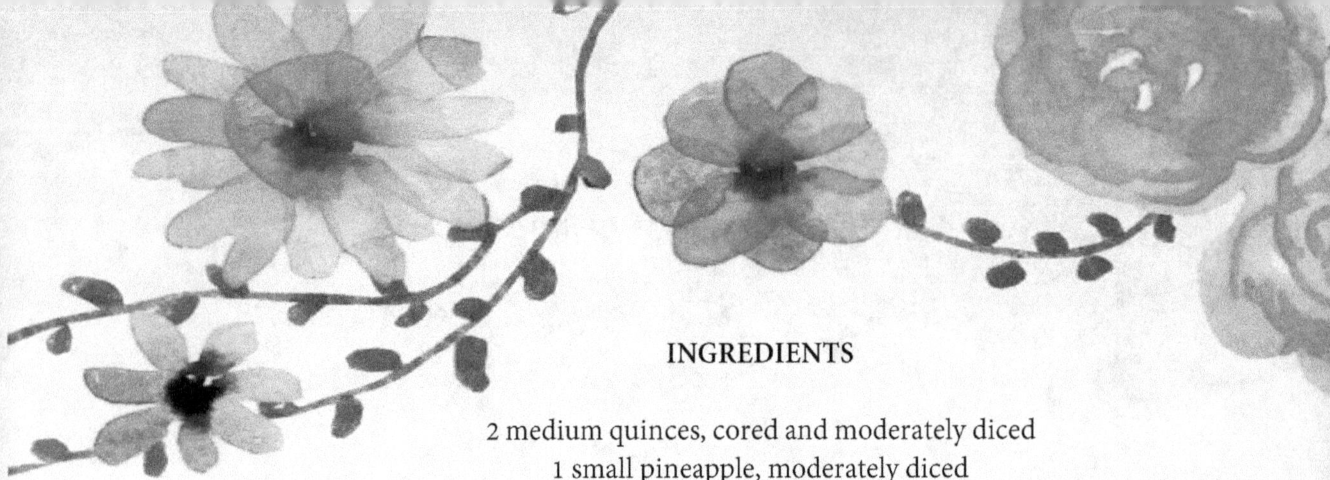

INGREDIENTS

2 medium quinces, cored and moderately diced
1 small pineapple, moderately diced
½ butternut squash, moderately diced
1 medium onion, diced small
½ teaspoon unrefined sea salt
3 tablespoons rice oil
1 tablespoon pure sesame oil *(from roasted seeds)*
¼ teaspoon mixed herbs of your choice *(See also page 6.)*

PREPARATION

1. Pour rice oil in a wok over medium-high heat.
2. Add quince and squash.
3. Stir-fry for at least 1 minute.
4. Add pineapple.
5. Stir-fry for at least 20 seconds.
6. Add onion.
7. Stir-fry for 20 seconds.
8. Add seasonings and salt.
9. Stir-fry for 1 minute.
10. Remove wok from heat.
11. Let it cool for 30 seconds.
12. Add sesame oil.
13. Stir all ingredients one more time.
14. Add chicken breast, cut into bite-size pieces, previously prepared as desired.
15. Stir one last time.
16. Serve hot, warm, or at room temperature.

You Matter!

1. Take four gorgeous pictures of your culinary result.

2. Write down your impressions of the recipe.

a. Did you like it?

____

b. Was it difficult?

____

c. Did you find all the ingredients?

____

d. Did you make any changes to the recipe to better suit your dietary needs?

____

____

e. Will you cook it again?

____

f. Will you share it with your family and friends?

____

g. How did it make your body feel?

____

____

h. How were you feeling before cooking the recipe?

____

____

i. How were you feeling after eating the culinary result?

____

____

TRUFFLES CHAMELEON

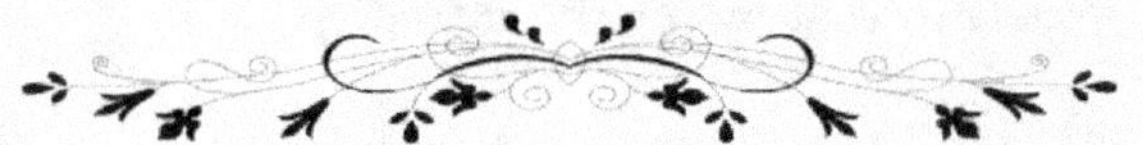

Here is a deeply indulgent dish made from three healthy ingredients. It is both therapeutic and nourishing, so both your body and your mind will thank you for your culinary choice.

You can also binge on these sweets when you are worrying about your future.

Type of Meal	Snack
	Dessert
Type of Dish	Lacto-Ovo-Vegetarian
	Non-Vegetarian
Preparation Time	Approximately 10 minutes
	Approximately 30 minutes, refrigeration time
Cooking Time	Approximately 20 minutes
Servings	15-20 pieces
The AilamA® Cookbook advises You	For this recipe, you can use any type of organic dates you can easily find.
	In case you find the mixture too sticky to roll, coat your hands in carob powder.

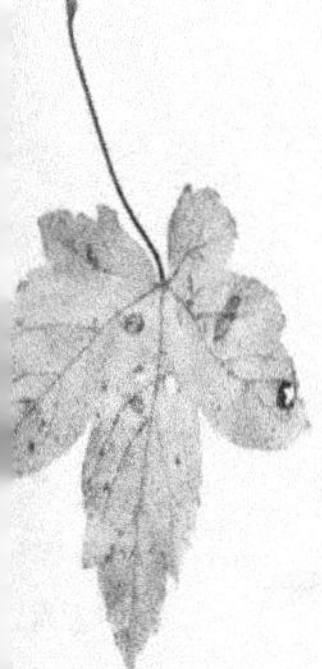

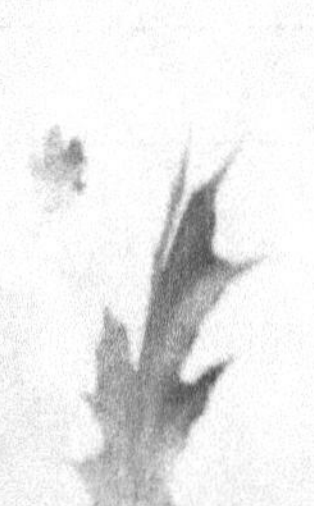

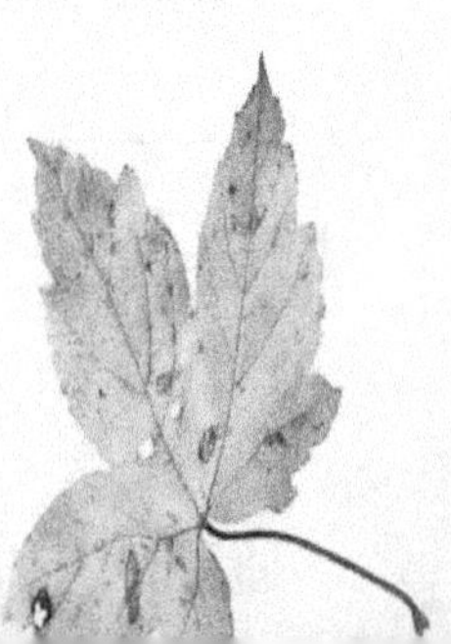

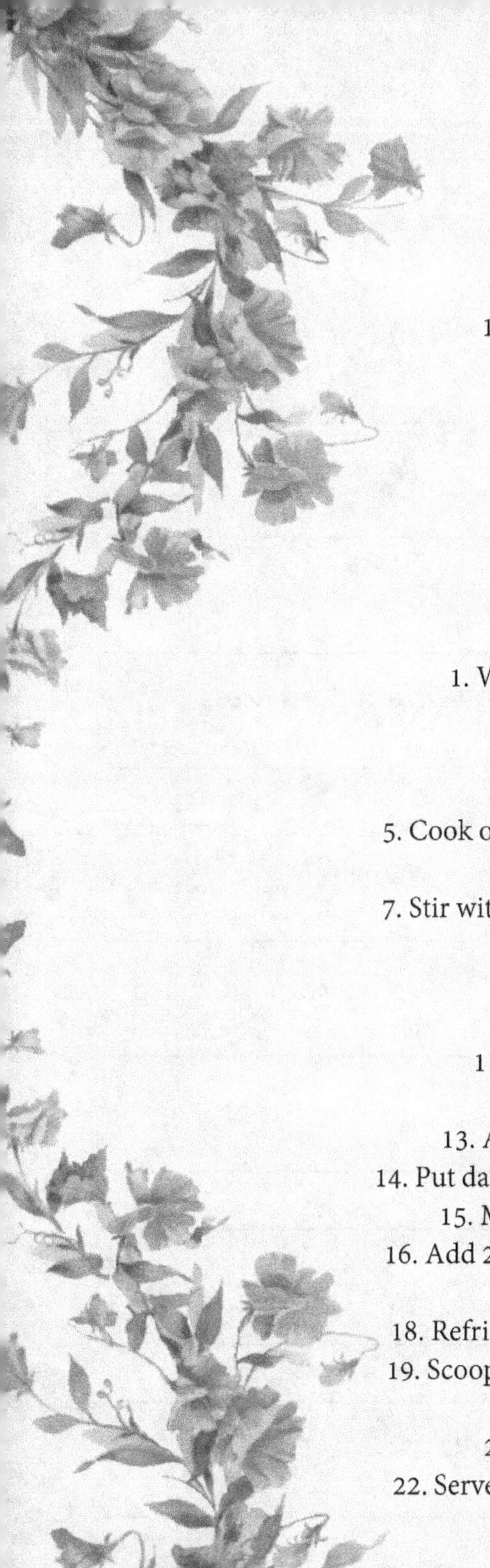

INGREDIENTS

3 cups organic barley grains *(pearled)*
3 cups spring water
1 small cup organic dates of your choice
½ small cup organic carob powder
Pinch of unrefined salt

PREPARATION

1. Wash and rinse barley thoroughly.
2. Add 3 cups of water.
3. Bring to a boil.
4. Let it boil for 30 seconds.
5. Cook over low heat until textured, not mushy.
6. Take out the white scum.
7. Stir with a spoon from time to time. *(optional)*
8. Remove from heat.
9. Add salt.
10. Mix well.
11. Cover with lid for 5 minutes.
12. Remove lid.
13. Allow to cool at room temperature.
14. Put dates and cooked barley in a blender bowl.
15. Mix ingredients into a thick cream.
16. Add 2 teaspoons of carob powder. *(optional)*
17. Mix until well combined.
18. Refrigerate batter for 30 minutes. *(optional)*
19. Scoop mixture into teaspoon-sized mounds.
20. Roll mounds into balls.
21. Coat balls in carob powder.
22. Serve cold, frozen, or at room temperature.

You Matter!

1. Take four gorgeous pictures of your culinary result.

2. Write down your impressions of the recipe.

a. Did you like it?

____

b. Was it difficult?

____

c. Did you find all the ingredients?

____

d. Did you make any changes to the recipe to better suit your dietary needs?

____

____

e. Will you cook it again?

____

f. Will you share it with your family and friends?

____

g. How did it make your body feel?

____

____

h. How were you feeling before cooking the recipe?

____

____

i. How were you feeling after eating the culinary result?

____

____

The Recipe of Week 19
LEEK WOK

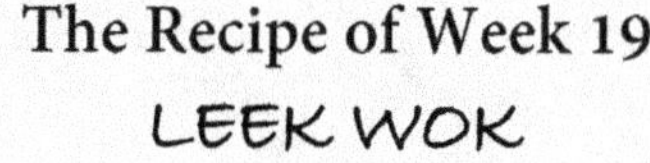
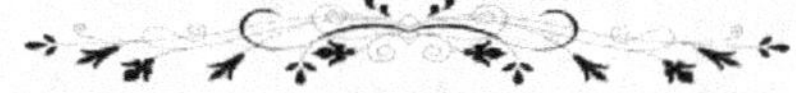

Here is yet another way of combining healthy vegetables in a tasty wok dish that is part of your culinary project 365. It can also be a perfect treat for the times when you can come home from work much earlier than usual.

Type of Meal	Main Course
	Lunch
	Dinner
Type of Dish	Vegetarian
	Non-Vegetarian
Preparation Time	Approximately 10 minutes
Cooking Time	Approximately 5 minutes
Servings	3
The AilamA® Cookbook advises You	This dish also goes well with chicken, turkey, or venison.

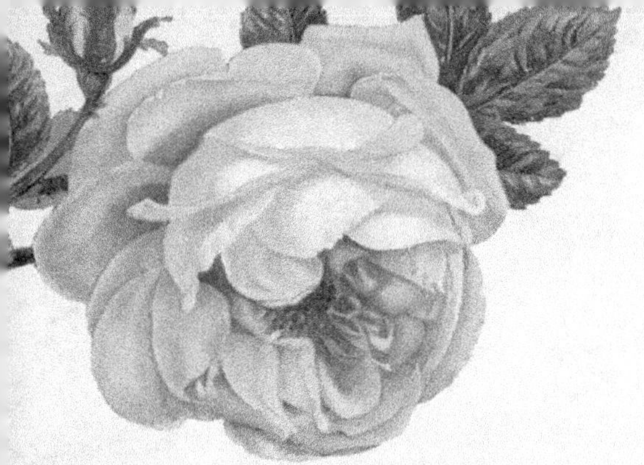

INGREDIENTS

2 large leeks, moderately sliced
2 medium bell peppers, sliced lengthwise, then halved crosswise
2 medium carrots, sliced lengthwise, then cut on the diagonal
1 handful dill, finely chopped
½ teaspoon unrefined sea salt
3 tablespoons rice oil
1 teaspoon mixed herbs of your choice *(See also page 6.)*
Beef, previously prepared as desired,
then cut into bite-size pieces *(non-vegetarian dish)*

PREPARATION

1. Pour rice oil in a wok over medium-high heat.
2. Add carrots.
3. Stir-fry for at least 1 minute.
4. Add pepper and leek.
5. Stir-fry for at least 1 minute.
6. Add dill, seasonings, and salt.
7. Stir-fry for 1 minute.
8. Remove wok from heat.
9. Let it cool for 1 minute.
10. Add beef. *(non-vegetarian dish)*
11. Stir one last time.
12. Serve hot, warm, or at room temperature.

You Matter!

1. Take four gorgeous pictures of your culinary result.

2. Write down your impressions of the recipe.

a. Did you like it?

____

b. Was it difficult?

____

c. Did you find all the ingredients?

____

d. Did you make any changes to the recipe to better suit your dietary needs?

____

____

e. Will you cook it again?

____

f. Will you share it with your family and friends?

____

g. How did it make your body feel?

____

____

h. How were you feeling before cooking the recipe?

____

____

i. How were you feeling after eating the culinary result?

____

____

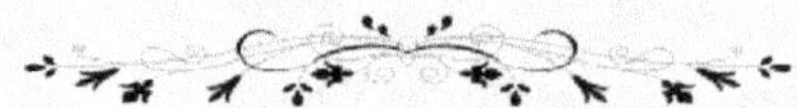

Here is a delicious wok with broccoli and other nutritious vegetables, a real energy booster.
You can also cook it in honor of all the good and kind people in the world, you included.

Type of Meal	Main Course Lunch
Type of Dish	Vegetarian Non-Vegetarian
Preparation Time	Approximately 10 minutes
Cooking Time	Approximately 10 minutes
Servings	4
The AilamA® Cookbook advises You	Broccoli sprouts are even denser in nutrients than mature broccoli. Broccoli seeds can germinate in a day or two. A teaspoon of germinated broccoli seeds a day can be enough for a mature person to maintain good health.

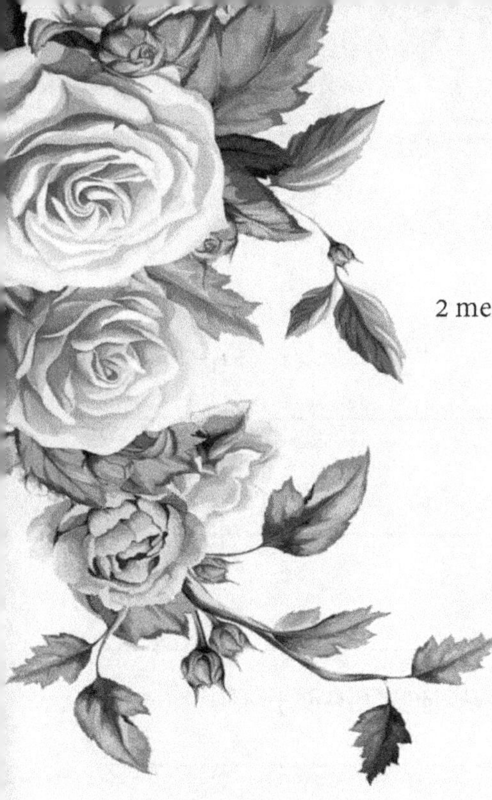

INGREDIENTS

1 large parsnip, cut into moderate chunks
½ medium celery root, cut into moderate chunks
2 medium sweet red peppers sliced lengthwise, then halved crosswise
¼ medium buttercup squash, moderately diced
1 medium quince, moderately diced
2 medium onions, sliced in full rings
4 handfuls broccoli florets, washed and cut in halves
3 cloves garlic, chopped
1 teaspoon unrefined sea salt
3 tablespoons rice oil
2 teaspoons mixed herbs of your choice *(See also page 6.)*
Meat of your choice, prepared as desired,
then cut into bite-size pieces *(non-vegetarian dish)*

PREPARATION

1. Pour rice oil in a wok over medium-high heat.
2. Add parsnip and celery.
3. Stir-fry for at least 1 minute.
4. Add pepper, quince, broccoli, and squash.
5. Stir-fry for at least 1 minute.
6. Add onion.
7. Stir-fry for at least 1 minute.
8. Add seasonings and salt.
9. Stir-fry for 30 seconds.
10. Remove wok from heat.
11. Let it cool for 1 minute.
12. Add meat. *(non-vegetarian dish)*
13. Stir one last time.
14. Serve it hot, warm, or at room temperature.

You Matter!

1. Take four gorgeous pictures of your culinary result.

2. Write down your impressions of the recipe.

a. Did you like it?

____

b. Was it difficult?

____

c. Did you find all the ingredients?

____

d. Did you make any changes to the recipe to better suit your dietary needs?

____

____

e. Will you cook it again?

____

f. Will you share it with your family and friends?

____

g. How did it make your body feel?

____

____

h. How were you feeling before cooking the recipe?

____

____

i. How were you feeling after eating the culinary result?

____

____

The Recipe of Week 21
CHINA MIX

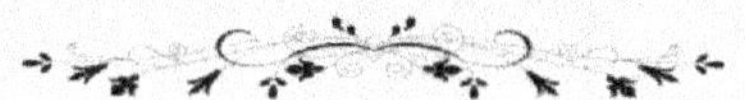

This delicious wok can be served when having guests, since it's quick to prepare and unforgettably flavored.

It can also be your culinary reminder of the universal power of harmonious interconnection.

Type of Meal	Main Course
	Lunch
Type of Dish	Vegetarian
	Non-Vegetarian
Preparation Time	Approximately 10 minutes
	Approximately 1 hour, soaking time
Cooking Time	Approximately 5 minutes
Servings	6
The AilamA® Cookbook advises You	Stir-frying is one of the best ways to cook rapidly with just a coat of oil.
	If in love with cooked food, this is exactly what you need.
	The ingredients keep their flavor as well as their crispy texture.

INGREDIENTS

½ large parsnip, cut into moderate chunks
½ medium celery root, cut into moderate chunks
2 medium sweet red peppers, sliced lengthwise then halved crosswise
¼ medium carrot, cut into moderate chunks
2 medium onions, sliced crosswise in full rings
3 handfuls broccoli florets, washed, cut into halves
2 handfuls green peas, washed
2 handfuls wood ear mushrooms,
previously soaked in water, washed, rinsed, wood ends removed
2 moderate bamboo shoots, halved lengthwise, then thinly sliced
6 cloves garlic, chopped
2 handfuls seaweed, previously soaked in water, washed and rinsed
1 teaspoon unrefined rock salt
3 tablespoons rice oil
1 tablespoon pure sesame oil *(from roasted seeds)*
2 teaspoons mixed herbs of your choice *(See also page 6.)*
Meat (chicken, hen, cock, beef, veal, venison), previously prepared as desired,
cut into bite-size pieces *(non-vegetarian dish)*

PREPARATION

1. Pour rice oil in a wok over medium-high heat.
2. Add parsnip, carrot, and celery.
3. Stir-fry for at least 1 minute.
4. Add pepper, mushrooms, bamboo shoots, broccoli, and peas.
5. Stir-fry for at least 1 minute.
6. Add onion, seaweed, and garlic.
7. Stir-fry for at least 30 seconds.
8. Add herbs and salt.
9. Remove wok from heat.
10. Let it cool for 1 minute.
11. Add meat. *(non-vegetarian dish)*
12. Add sesame oil.
13. Stir one last time.
14. Serve it hot, warm, or at room temperature.

You Matter!

1. Take four gorgeous pictures of your culinary result.

2. Write down your impressions of the recipe.

a. Did you like it?

____

b. Was it difficult?

____

c. Did you find all the ingredients?

____

d. Did you make any changes to the recipe to better suit your dietary needs?

____

____

e. Will you cook it again?

____

f. Will you share it with your family and friends?

____

g. How did it make your body feel?

____

____

h. How were you feeling before cooking the recipe?

____

____

i. How were you feeling after eating the culinary result?

____

____

MINTY BROWN CREAM

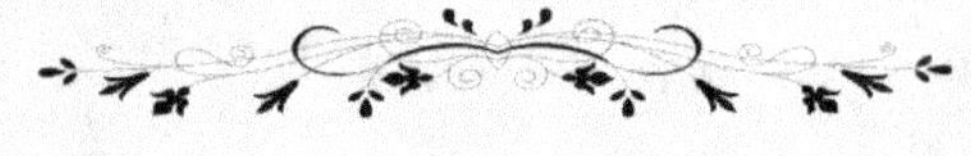

Here is an easy mint chocolate recipe to try during your culinary project 365.

You can also eat this refreshingly sweet dish whenever you feel sorry for other people, whether you know them personally or not.

Type of Meal	Dessert
	Snack
Type of Dish	Lacto-Ovo-Vegetarian
	Non-Vegetarian
Preparation Time	Approximately 1 minute
Cooking Time	Approximately 8 minutes
Servings	6
The AilamA® Cookbook advises You	Carob is the perfect cocoa replacer, with a distinct flavour and a nice texture when combined with melted butter. Keep in mind that carob creams can be runnier than their cocoa counterparts. *(See also page 50.)*

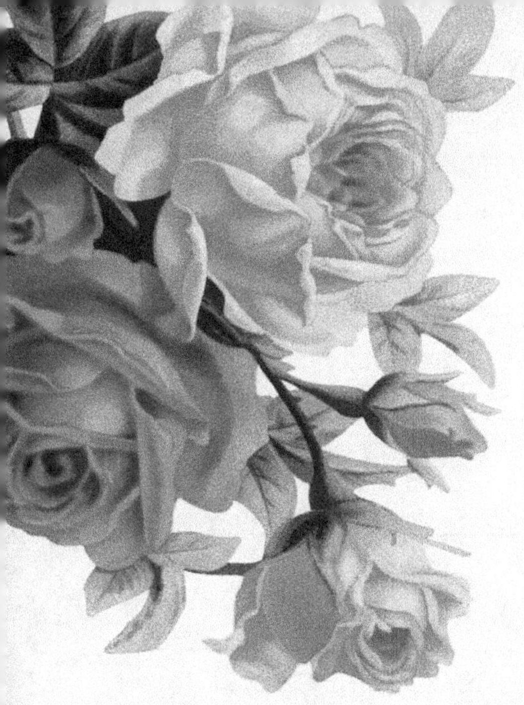

INGREDIENTS

1 egg
2 teaspoons coconut blossom sugar
2 tablespoons (clarified) butter
2 teaspoons cocoa powder *or* carob powder
½ teaspoon (germinated) flaxseeds
¼ teaspoon dried mint leaves, powdered
1 drop mint extract

PREPARATION

1. Mix egg with sugar in a pot.
2. Stir until blended.
3. Set pot in a bain-marie.
4. Add butter.
5. Stir until well blended and creamy.
6. Add cocoa or carob powder, flaxseeds, and mint powder.
7. Mix well for 1 minute or so.
8. Remove pot from heat.
9. Let it cool for 2 minutes.
10. Pierce cream with a toothpick.
11. Pour mint drop into hole.
12. Mix well.
13. Pour cream in a glass bowl.
14. Let it cool for 5 minutes.
15. Serve chilled or at room temperature.

You Matter!

1. Take four gorgeous pictures of your culinary result.

2. Write down your impressions of the recipe.

a. Did you like it?

____

b. Was it difficult?

____

c. Did you find all the ingredients?

____

d. Did you make any changes to the recipe to better suit your dietary needs?

____

____

e. Will you cook it again?

____

f. Will you share it with your family and friends?

____

g. How did it make your body feel?

____

____

h. How were you feeling before cooking the recipe?

____

____

i. How were you feeling after eating the culinary result?

____

____

POTATO & MUSHROOM STEW

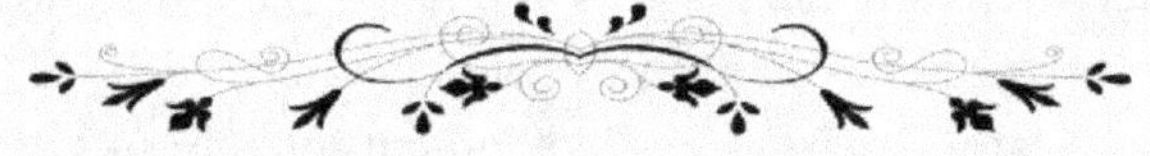

Here is a stew recipe packed with macronutrients to keep both vegetarians and non-vegetarians healthy.

You can also eat this stew when you feel angry because you have been treated unfairly at your workplace.

Type of Meal	Main Course Lunch Dinner
Type of Dish	Vegetarian Non-Vegetarian
Preparation Time	Approximately 15 minutes
Cooking Time	Approximately 60 minutes
Servings	8
The AilamA® Cookbook advises You	This stew contains no tomato juice or flour, so it makes a great dish even if you suffer from poor digestion, or if you are diabetic.

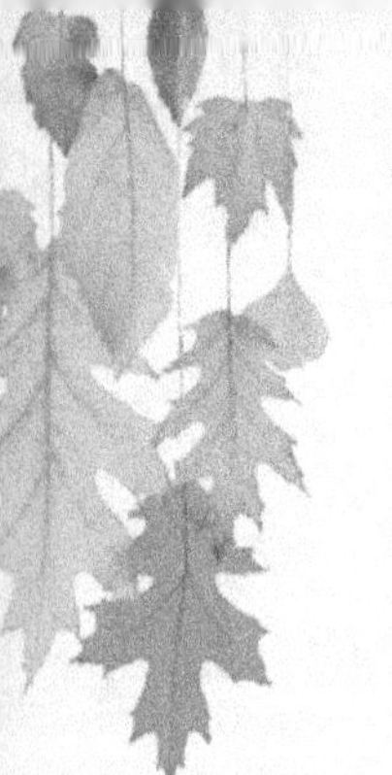

INGREDIENTS

2 large carrots, finely grated
1 small celery root, finely grated
1 saucerful fresh celery, stalks and leaves, roughly chopped
2 medium onions, roughly chopped
6 large potatoes, peeled and cut into chunks
2 handfuls mushrooms of your choice, roughly chopped
1 teaspoon unrefined rock salt
8 tablespoons extra virgin olive oil
8 cups spring water
8 cups beef stock/chicken broth *(non-vegetarian dish)*
2 teaspoons mixed herbs of your choice *(See also page 6.)*
2 saucerfuls beef or chicken breast, boiled and diced *(non-vegetarian dish)*

PREPARATION

1. Pour olive oil in a cauldron/deep pot over medium heat.
2. Add spring water.
Add beef stock/chicken broth. *(non-vegetarian dish)*
3. Add potatoes.
4. Occasionally, stir with wooden spoon.
5. Scrape the brown bits off the bottom of the cauldron, if any.
6. Cook until potatoes are halfway tender.
7. Add mushrooms and onion.
8. Stir from time to time.
9. Add beef/chicken breast. *(non-vegetarian dish)*
10. Let it simmer uncovered for 15 minutes.
11. Add carrots and celery root.
12. Let it simmer for 10 minutes.
13. Add celery stalks and leaves.
14. Let it simmer until done.
15. Remove cauldron from heat.
16. Add salt and herbs.
17. Stir one last time.
18. Serve it hot or warm.

You Matter!

1. Take four gorgeous pictures of your culinary result.

2. Write down your impressions of the recipe.

a. Did you like it?

____

b. Was it difficult?

____

c. Did you find all the ingredients?

____

d. Did you make any changes to the recipe to better suit your dietary needs?

____

____

e. Will you cook it again?

____

f. Will you share it with your family and friends?

____

g. How did it make your body feel?

____

____

h. How were you feeling before cooking the recipe?

____

____

i. How were you feeling after eating the culinary result?

____

____

CHOCO-DELIGHT

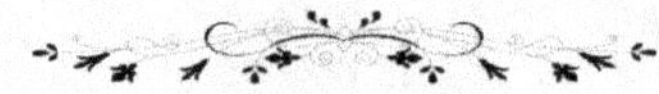

Here is an easy recipe that will keep you away from all the sweet shelf products, packed with ingredients you can't even pronounce.
You can also indulge yourself with this sweet dish when you feel pain at all the undeserved misfortunes in your life.

Type of Meal	Dessert
	Snack
Type of Dish	Lacto-Ovo-Vegetarian
	Non-Vegetarian
Preparation Time	Approximately 1 minute
Cooking Time	Approximately 4 minutes
Servings	6
The AilamA® Cookbook advises You	Chocolate creams can be sweet or bitter, runny or thick, depending on one's taste. You can adapt this recipe to your own taste by adding a larger amount of sweetener, more cocoa or carob powder, or even more water. The best way to decide is by tasting the cream from time to time.

INGREDIENTS

1 egg
2 teaspoons coconut blossom sugar
1 tablespoon clarified butter
2 teaspoons cocoa powder *or* carob powder
1 teaspoon sesame seeds

PREPARATION

1. Mix egg with sugar in a pot.
2. Stir until blended.
3. Set pot in a bain-marie.
4. Add butter.
5. Stir until well blended and creamy.
6. Add cocoa or carob powder.
7. Mix well for 1 minute or so.
8. Remove pot from heat.
9. Let it cool for 2 minutes.
10. Pour content in small pots.
11. Sprinkle with sesame seeds on top.
12. Serve it warm, cold, or frozen.

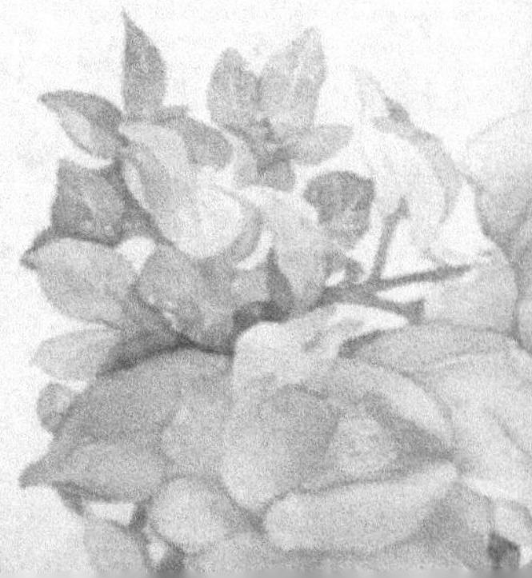

You Matter!

1. Take four gorgeous pictures of your culinary result.

2. Write down your impressions of the recipe.

a. Did you like it?

____

b. Was it difficult?

____

c. Did you find all the ingredients?

____

d. Did you make any changes to the recipe to better suit your dietary needs?

____

____

e. Will you cook it again?

____

f. Will you share it with your family and friends?

____

g. How did it make your body feel?

____

____

h. How were you feeling before cooking the recipe?

____

____

i. How were you feeling after eating the culinary result?

____

____

VEGGIE STEW

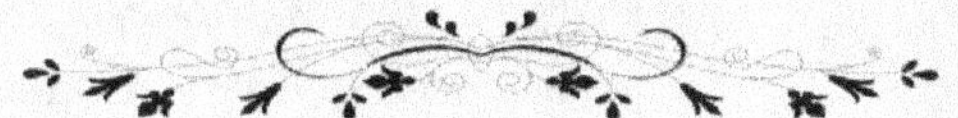

Clay or ceramic cookware is an excellent choice for slow cooking in the oven, and this recipe is a case in point.

This delicious stew can also accompany your musing about the possibility of doing something audacious, like starting your own business or cutting your bangs at home.

Type of Meal	Main Course
	Lunch
	Supper
Type of Dish	Vegetarian
	Non-Vegetarian
Preparation Time	Approximately 5 minutes
Cooking Time	Approximately 1 hour
Servings	6
The AilamA® Cookbook advises You	Cook food in clay pots, but don't store it in them, since it can get a strange taste and smell from the clay.

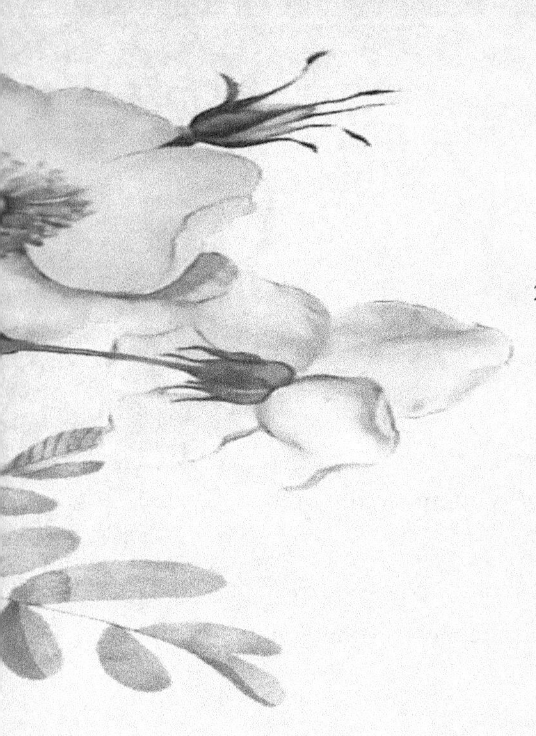

INGREDIENTS

1 large zucchini, moderately cut
2 large sweet red peppers, moderately cut
2 handfuls broccoli florets, halved
1 cup green peas, washed
1 handful string beans, washed, halved
2 celery stalks, moderately sliced
1 handful oyster mushrooms
1 red onion, moderately diced
6 cloves garlic, peeled and crushed
½ celery root, moderately diced
1 large carrot, moderately diced
3 tablespoons rice oil
2 teaspoons unrefined sea salt
2 teaspoons mixed herbs of your choice *(See also page 6.)*
1 cup spring water
Meat of your choice, prepared as desired, bite-size pieces *(non-vegetarian dish)*

PREPARATION

1. Put water, vegetables, salt, and herbs into a clay baking pot.
2. Cover with lid.
3. Turn oven to 160 degrees C (320 degrees F).
4. Cook in oven for approximately 1 hour.
5. Let it cool for 2 minutes.
6. Add oil while stirring the contents.
7. Add meat. *(non-vegetarian dish)*
8. Stir one last time.
9. Serve hot, warm, or at room temperature.

You Matter!

1. Take four gorgeous pictures of your culinary result.

2. Write down your impressions of the recipe.

a. Did you like it?

____

b. Was it difficult?

____

c. Did you find all the ingredients?

____

d. Did you make any changes to the recipe to better suit your dietary needs?

____

____

e. Will you cook it again?

____

f. Will you share it with your family and friends?

____

g. How did it make your body feel?

____

____

h. How were you feeling before cooking the recipe?

____

____

i. How were you feeling after eating the culinary result?

____

____

BAKED MEAT

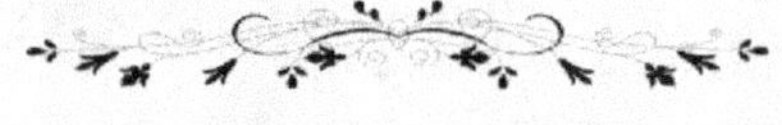

Use the magic clay pot for all your meats. You'll certainly taste the difference. You can also add baked meat to your meals whenever you can't help feeling jealous of what others have and you don't.

Type of Meal	Main Course Lunch
Type of Dish	Non-Vegetarian
Preparation Time	Approximately 5 minutes Approximately 4 hours, baking time
Cooking Time	Approximately 4 hours
Servings	4
The AilamA® Cookbook advises You	You can put veggies and anything else you like in the baking pot together with your chicken, turkey, or hen. Just make sure you will add them 25 minutes before baking time ends.

INGREDIENTS

Beef *(3 hours, baking time)*
Venison *(4 hours, baking time)*
Organic chicken *(1½ hours, baking time)*
Hen *or* cock *(2½ -3 hours, baking time)*
Rabbit *or* hare *(2½ -3 hours, baking time)*
Unrefined rock salt
Dried herbs of your choice *(See also page 6.)*
Fresh herbs as desired

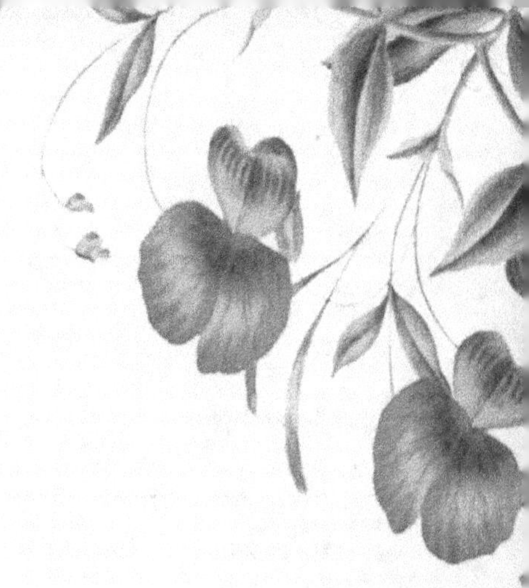

PREPARATION

1. Put meat or poultry in a pot.
2. Bring it to a boil.
3. Boil it for 10 minutes.
4. Take off all scum.
5. Put meat or poultry in a baking pot.
6. Add spring water to cover it half.
7. Add herbs and salt in water.
8. Rub meat with herbs and salt.
9. Close with lid.
10. Set the oven temperature to minimum.
11. Bake in oven as recommended. *(See also page 4.)*
12. Serve hot, warm, or at room temperature.

You Matter!

1. Take four gorgeous pictures of your culinary result.

2. Write down your impressions of the recipe.

a. Did you like it?

____

b. Was it difficult?

____

c. Did you find all the ingredients?

____

d. Did you make any changes to the recipe to better suit your dietary needs?

____

____

e. Will you cook it again?

____

f. Will you share it with your family and friends?

____

g. How did it make your body feel?

____

____

h. How were you feeling before cooking the recipe?

____

____

i. How were you feeling after eating the culinary result?

____

____

CEDAR NUT DRESSING

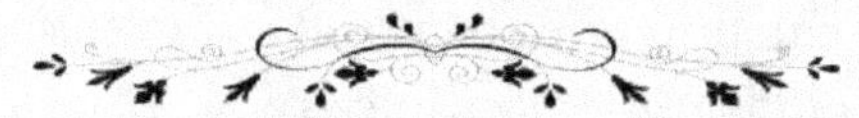

Here is a tasty dressing to combine with any food you like.
You can also use it with your meals whenever you feel it's so hard to do things alone.

Type of Meal	Lunch
	Supper
	Snack
Type of Dish	Vegetarian
	Non-Vegetarian
Preparation Time	Approximately 5 minutes
Cooking Time	0 minutes
Servings	2½ cups
The AilamA® Cookbook advises You	You can tweak this recipe by changing the type of nuts or seeds. If you use walnuts or almonds, blend them until coarsely chopped.

INGREDIENTS

½ cup extra virgin olive oil
½ cup unrefined hemp oil
1 moderate lemon, juiced
2 tablespoons fresh parsley, washed and finely chopped
½ cup cedar nuts, raw, germinated, or roasted
¼ teaspoon ground ginger
¼ teaspoon unrefined rock salt
¼ teaspoon mixed herbs of your choice *(See also page 6.)*

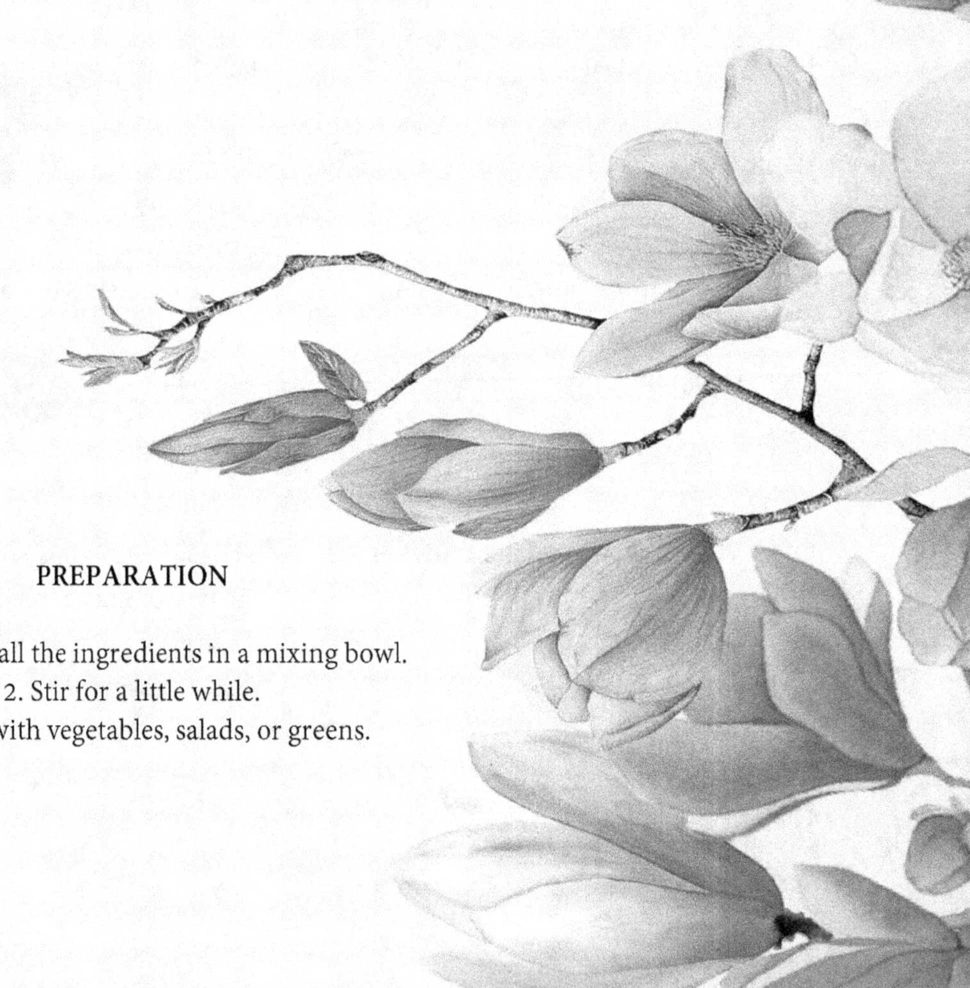

PREPARATION

1. Combine all the ingredients in a mixing bowl.
2. Stir for a little while.
3. Serve with vegetables, salads, or greens.

You Matter!

1. Take four gorgeous pictures of your culinary result.

2. Write down your impressions of the recipe.

a. Did you like it?

____

b. Was it difficult?

____

c. Did you find all the ingredients?

____

d. Did you make any changes to the recipe to better suit your dietary needs?

____

____

e. Will you cook it again?

____

f. Will you share it with your family and friends?

____

g. How did it make your body feel?

____

____

h. How were you feeling before cooking the recipe?

____

____

i. How were you feeling after eating the culinary result?

____

____

SEAWEED SALAD

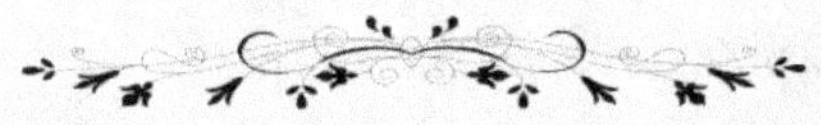

Here is a simple salad that has the power to revitalize your hormones.

Your can also make this dish your celebratory food when you think that fortune has smiled on you.

Type of Meal	Salad
	Side Dish
Type of Dish	Vegetarian
	Non-Vegetarian
Preparation Time	Approximately 5 minutes
	Approximately 30 minutes, soaking time
Cooking Time	0 minutes
Servings	4
The AilamA® Cookbook advises You	You should use a pair of scissors to cut the seaweed into smaller pieces before soaking. It's more difficult to do it afterward. Instead of almonds, you can use regular lettuce, or you can use them together.

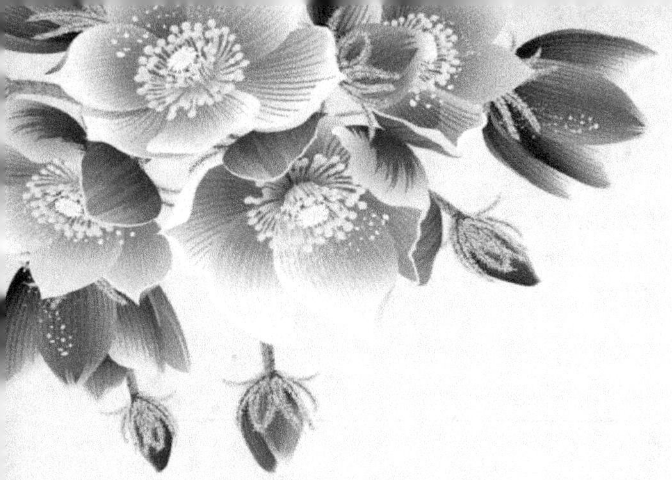

INGREDIENTS

½ pack dried seaweed *(kelp, wakame, or dulse)*
4 tablespoons extra virgin olive oil
½ cup (germinated) almonds, coarsely ground
3 cloves garlic, crushed and peeled
1 moderate lemon, juiced
¼ teaspoon unrefined rock salt

PREPARATION

1. Soak seaweed in spring water for 30 minutes.
2. Wash and rinse thoroughly.
3. Transfer to a mixing bowl.
4. Add oil, salt, almonds, lemon juice, and garlic.
5. Mix well.
6. Serve with meats or as a dish of itself.

You Matter!

1. Take four gorgeous pictures of your culinary result.

2. Write down your impressions of the recipe.

a. Did you like it?

____

b. Was it difficult?

____

c. Did you find all the ingredients?

____

d. Did you make any changes to the recipe to better suit your dietary needs?

____

____

e. Will you cook it again?

____

f. Will you share it with your family and friends?

____

g. How did it make your body feel?

____

____

h. How were you feeling before cooking the recipe?

____

____

i. How were you feeling after eating the culinary result?

____

____

RUBY SOUR-SWEET

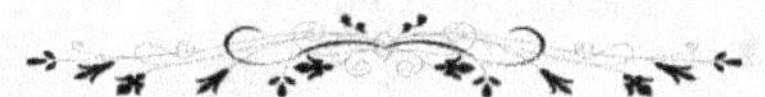

Did you know that preserves could be prepared entirely without added sugar? Here is the recipe for the healthiest version of all supermarket preserves.

You can also indulge yourself with this therapeutic preserve spread on spelt flatbread whenever you are alone and in dire need of a warm hug.

Type of Meal	Snack
	Dessert
Type of Dish	Vegetarian
	Non-Vegetarian
Preparation Time	Approximately 10 minutes
Cooking Time	Approximately 30 minutes
Servings	4 small jars
The AilamA® Cookbook advises You	Sugar-free preserves allow the natural sweet-sourness of the fruit to be fully savored. You can boil sugar-free preserves for longer than 1 hour to turn them into healthy jams. *(See also page 186.)*

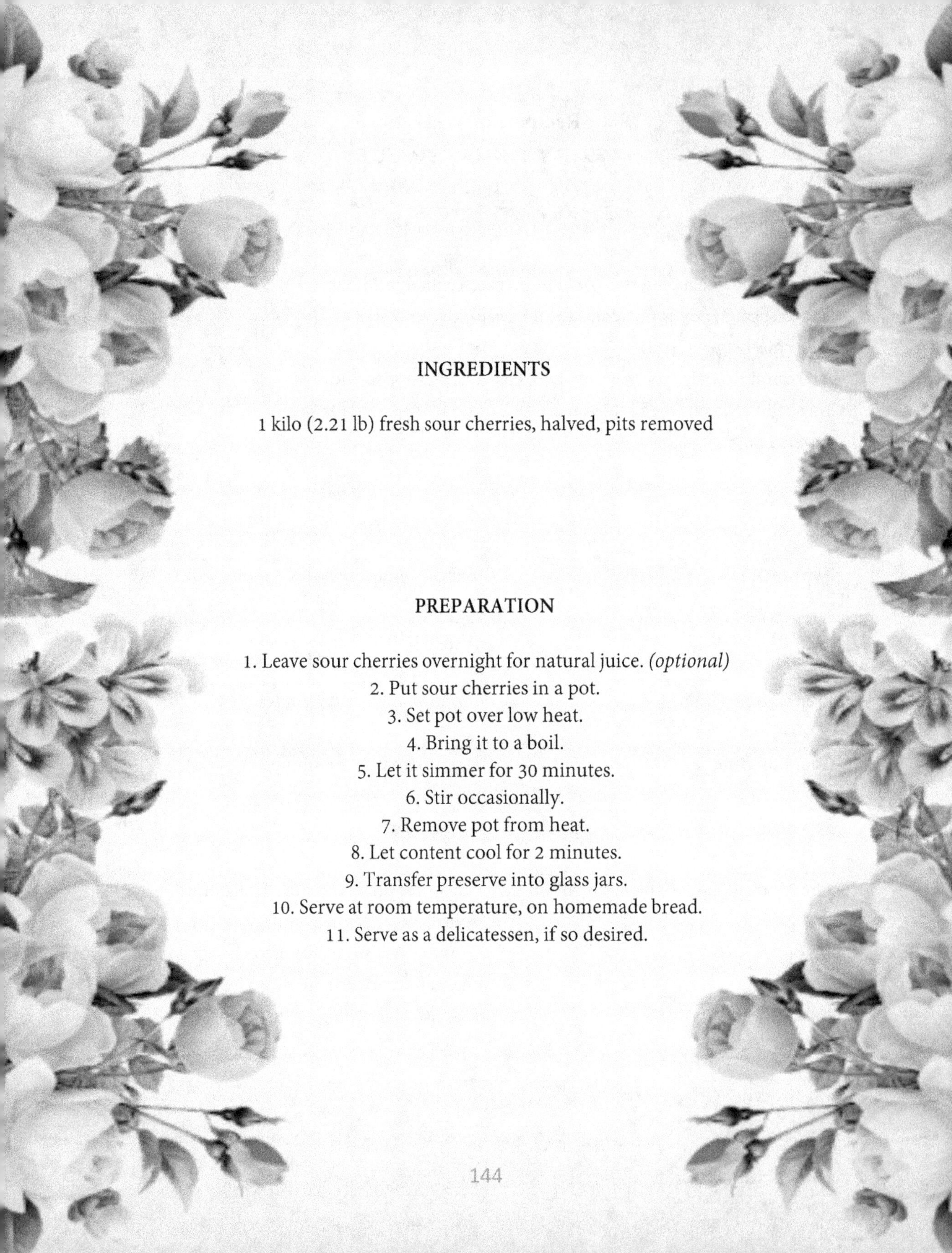

INGREDIENTS

1 kilo (2.21 lb) fresh sour cherries, halved, pits removed

PREPARATION

1. Leave sour cherries overnight for natural juice. *(optional)*
2. Put sour cherries in a pot.
3. Set pot over low heat.
4. Bring it to a boil.
5. Let it simmer for 30 minutes.
6. Stir occasionally.
7. Remove pot from heat.
8. Let content cool for 2 minutes.
9. Transfer preserve into glass jars.
10. Serve at room temperature, on homemade bread.
11. Serve as a delicatessen, if so desired.

You Matter!

1. Take four gorgeous pictures of your culinary result.

2. Write down your impressions of the recipe.

a. Did you like it?

____

b. Was it difficult?

____

c. Did you find all the ingredients?

____

d. Did you make any changes to the recipe to better suit your dietary needs?

____

____

e. Will you cook it again?

____

f. Will you share it with your family and friends?

____

g. How did it make your body feel?

____

____

h. How were you feeling before cooking the recipe?

____

____

i. How were you feeling after eating the culinary result?

____

____

CHOCO-EXOTIQUE

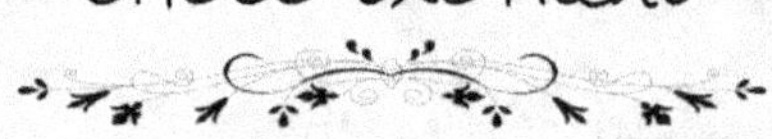

Here is a recipe with unpredictable taste combinations.
You can also binge on it whenever you feel you can achieve all of your goals with the greatest of ease.

Type of Meal	Dessert Snack
Type of Dish	Lacto-Ovo-Vegetarian Non-Vegetarian
Preparation Time	Approximately 1 minute
Cooking Time	Approximately 8 minutes
Servings	6
The AilamA® Cookbook advises You	Hemp seeds don't need to be soaked in water. They come in vacuum sealer bags because of their oily texture.

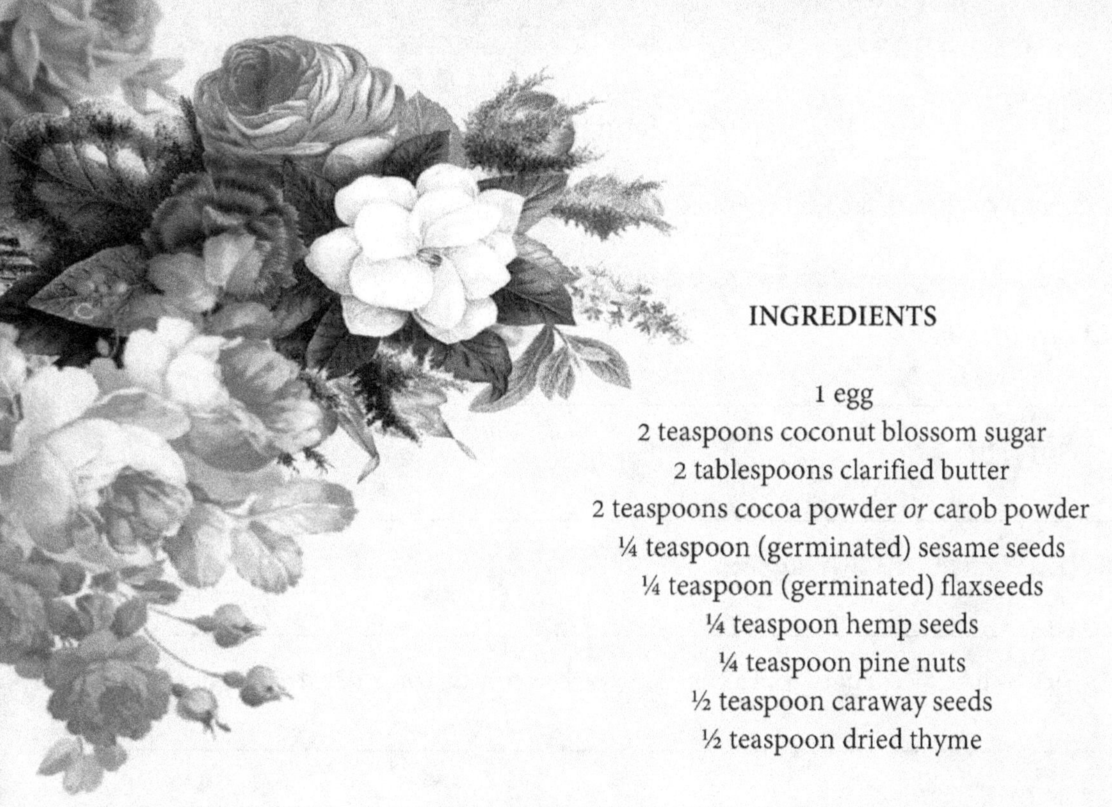

INGREDIENTS

1 egg
2 teaspoons coconut blossom sugar
2 tablespoons clarified butter
2 teaspoons cocoa powder *or* carob powder
¼ teaspoon (germinated) sesame seeds
¼ teaspoon (germinated) flaxseeds
¼ teaspoon hemp seeds
¼ teaspoon pine nuts
½ teaspoon caraway seeds
½ teaspoon dried thyme

PREPARATION

1. Mix egg with sugar in a pot.
2. Stir until blended.
3. Set pot in a bain-marie.
4. Add butter, sesame seeds, flaxseeds, hemp seeds, and pine seeds.
5. Stir until well blended and creamy.
6. Add cocoa or carob powder.
7. Mix well for 1 minute or so.
8. Remove pot from heat.
9. Let it cool for 2 minutes.
10. Pour content in 2 small pots.
11. Sprinkle one pot with caraway seeds on top.
12. Sprinkle other pot with dried thyme on top.
13. Serve it chilled or at room temperature.

You Matter!

1. Take four gorgeous pictures of your culinary result.

2. Write down your impressions of the recipe.

a. Did you like it?

____

b. Was it difficult?

____

c. Did you find all the ingredients?

____

d. Did you make any changes to the recipe to better suit your dietary needs?

____

____

e. Will you cook it again?

____

f. Will you share it with your family and friends?

____

g. How did it make your body feel?

____

____

h. How were you feeling before cooking the recipe?

____

____

i. How were you feeling after eating the culinary result?

____

____

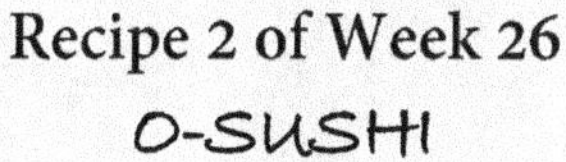

O-SUSHI

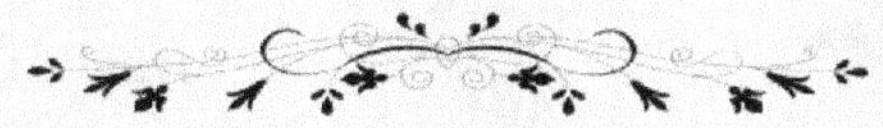

Here is a rapid sushi recipe that combines no starches with fish, which makes it ideal for all those who want to lose weight.

It is also ideal for the full-moon nights when you can't sleep and want something exotic to eat.

Type of Meal	Main Course
	Appetizer
	Snack
Type of Dish	Pesco-Ovo-Vegetarian
	Non-Vegetarian
Preparation Time	Approximately 10 minutes
	Approximately 20 minutes, boiling time
Cooking Time	Approximately 20 minutes
Servings	4
The AilamA® Cookbook advises You	If you are not familiar with rolling sushi, please first read the instructions on the pack of nori seaweed sheets.

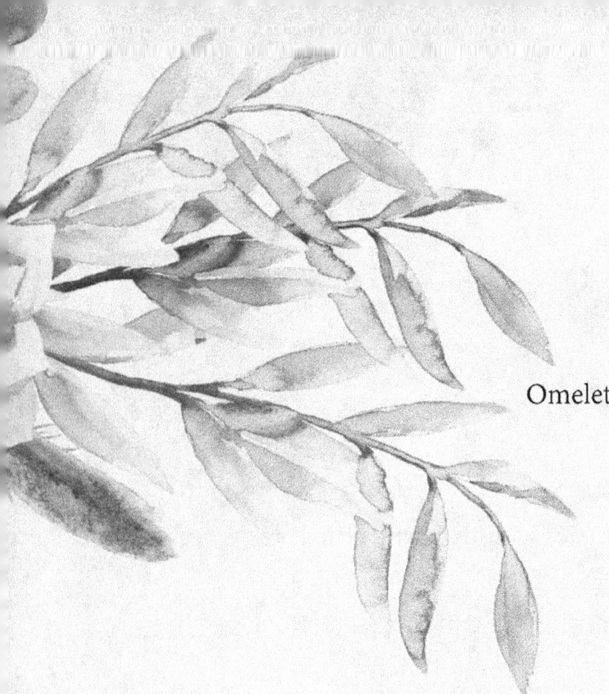

INGREDIENTS

2 sheets nori seaweed
Omelet of 1 egg, 2 egg whites, rice oil, and chopped fresh parsley
1 large strip tuna fish, canned in water
2 long strips red pepper
1 lemon, juiced
1 strip green salad
Pinch of salt
1 tablespoon (germinated) sesame seeds *(optional)*
Grated horseradish, pickled *(optional)*
or
Fresh ginger, grated *(optional)*

PREPARATION

1. Position nori seaweed on a bamboo mat.
2. Place cold omelette on nori.
3. Add all ingredients above.
4. Sprinkle with salt and lemon.
5. Roll to form sushi.
6. Slice with a sharp knife.
7. Serve with pickled horseradish or fresh ginger on top.
8. Serve with sesame seeds on top.

You Matter!

1. Take four gorgeous pictures of your culinary result.

2. Write down your impressions of the recipe.

a. Did you like it?

____

b. Was it difficult?

____

c. Did you find all the ingredients?

____

d. Did you make any changes to the recipe to better suit your dietary needs?

____

____

e. Will you cook it again?

____

f. Will you share it with your family and friends?

____

g. How did it make your body feel?

____

____

h. How were you feeling before cooking the recipe?

____

____

i. How were you feeling after eating the culinary result?

____

____

RICE BOOST

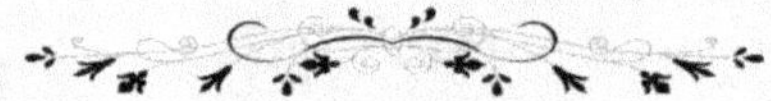

Rice can be eaten in different healthy combinations. Here is how it can be prepared for sushi or veggie dishes.

You can also eat it by itself before exercising. As its name says, it will boost your natural energy and recharge your batteries.

Type of Meal	Lunch
	Dinner
Type of Dish	Vegetarian
	Non-Vegetarian
Preparation Time	Approximately 5 minutes
Cooking Time	Approximately 20 minutes
Servings	4
The AilamA® Cookbook advises You	Millet and quinoa can also be cooked by following the same directions. *(See also pages 48 and 61.)*

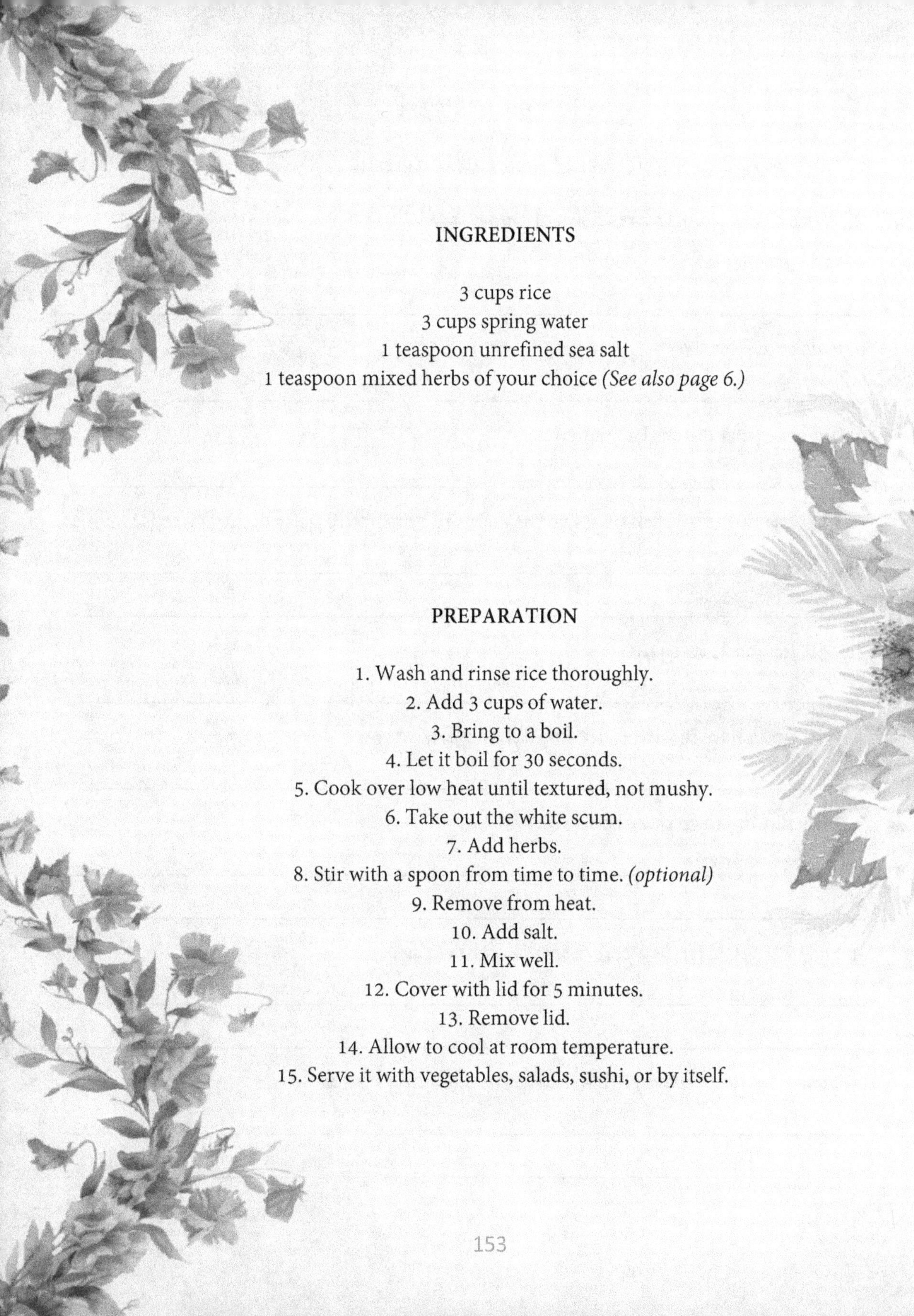

INGREDIENTS

3 cups rice
3 cups spring water
1 teaspoon unrefined sea salt
1 teaspoon mixed herbs of your choice *(See also page 6.)*

PREPARATION

1. Wash and rinse rice thoroughly.
2. Add 3 cups of water.
3. Bring to a boil.
4. Let it boil for 30 seconds.
5. Cook over low heat until textured, not mushy.
6. Take out the white scum.
7. Add herbs.
8. Stir with a spoon from time to time. *(optional)*
9. Remove from heat.
10. Add salt.
11. Mix well.
12. Cover with lid for 5 minutes.
13. Remove lid.
14. Allow to cool at room temperature.
15. Serve it with vegetables, salads, sushi, or by itself.

You Matter!

1. Take four gorgeous pictures of your culinary result.

2. Write down your impressions of the recipe.

a. Did you like it?

____

b. Was it difficult?

____

c. Did you find all the ingredients?

____

d. Did you make any changes to the recipe to better suit your dietary needs?

____

____

e. Will you cook it again?

____

f. Will you share it with your family and friends?

____

g. How did it make your body feel?

____

____

h. How were you feeling before cooking the recipe?

____

____

i. How were you feeling after eating the culinary result?

____

____

HONEY-DELIGHT

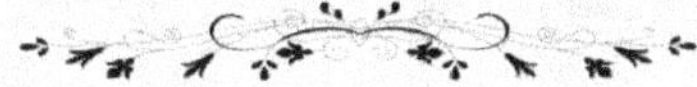

If you need a rapid sweet snack to help you get through the day, here is one that you'll love.

Also, don't hesitate to eat it in the moments when you don't feel loved or appreciated.

Type of Meal	Dessert
	Snack
Type of Dish	Vegetarian
	Raw Vegan
	Non-Vegetarian
Preparation Time	Approximately 1 minute
	Approximately 3 hours, soaking time
Cooking Time	0 minutes
Servings	4
The AilamA® Cookbook advises You	Make sure raw honey is organic.

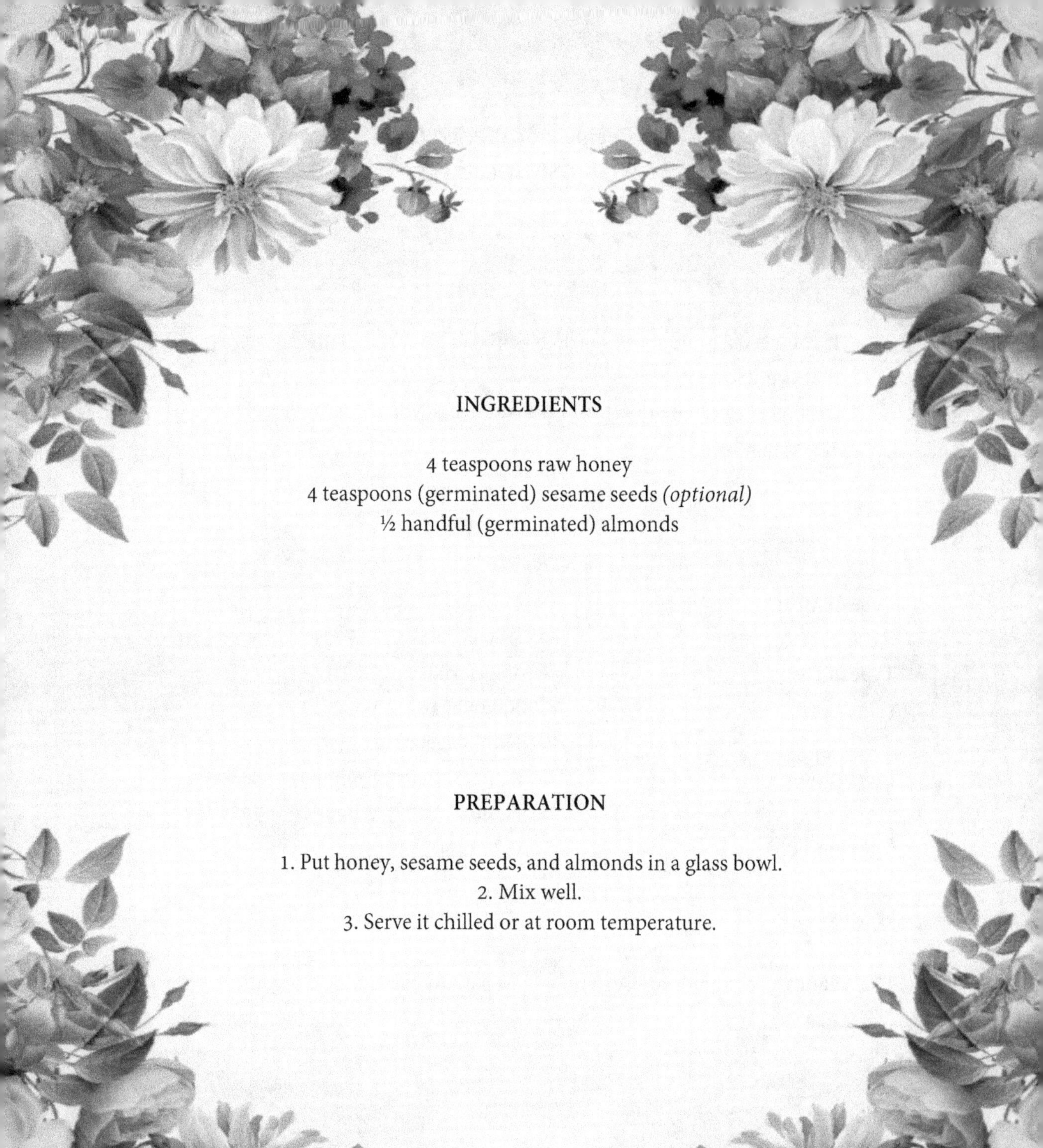

INGREDIENTS

4 teaspoons raw honey
4 teaspoons (germinated) sesame seeds *(optional)*
½ handful (germinated) almonds

PREPARATION

1. Put honey, sesame seeds, and almonds in a glass bowl.
2. Mix well.
3. Serve it chilled or at room temperature.

You Matter!

1. Take four gorgeous pictures of your culinary result.

2. Write down your impressions of the recipe.

a. Did you like it?

____

b. Was it difficult?

____

c. Did you find all the ingredients?

____

d. Did you make any changes to the recipe to better suit your dietary needs?

____

____

e. Will you cook it again?

____

f. Will you share it with your family and friends?

____

g. How did it make your body feel?

____

____

h. How were you feeling before cooking the recipe?

____

____

i. How were you feeling after eating the culinary result?

____

____

VEGGIE WHITE DELIGHT

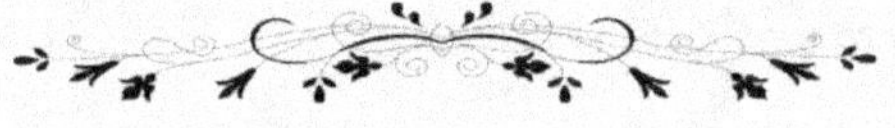
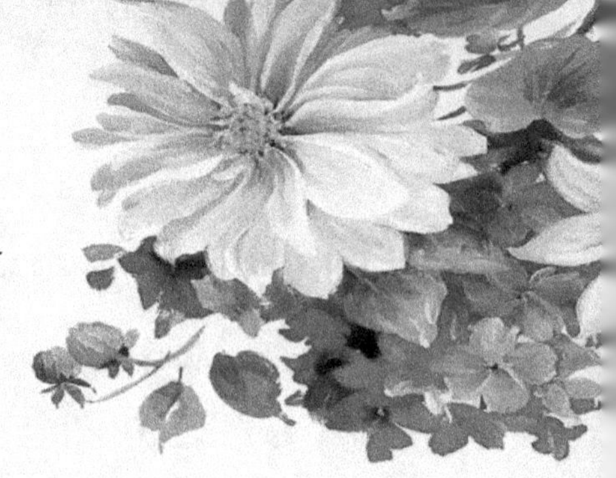

Here is a rapid vegetable stew for lunch or dinner. Enjoy!
You can also share it with a new friend the first time they drop in on you on their way home from work.

Type of Meal	Main Course Side Dish
Type of Dish	Vegetarian Non-Vegetarian
Preparation Time	Approximately 10 minutes Approximately 15 minutes, boiling time Approximately 1 hour, soaking time
Cooking Time	Approximately 5 minutes
Servings	4
The AilamA® Cookbook advises You	Starches should be combined with neither meats nor seafood, since they digest at different rates and could therefore cause digestive problems. However, if you feel like adding some meat leftovers, then go ahead. Also, if you want the white sauce thicker or runnier, add some more flour or water. Just be creative and remember to taste it from time to time.

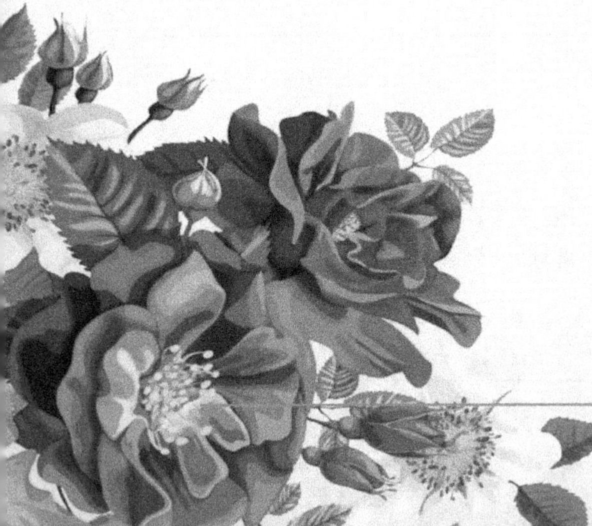

INGREDIENTS

2 large carrots, cut into moderate chunks
1 medium sweet red pepper sliced lengthwise, then halved crosswise
1 handful green beans, previously boiled, halved
1 cup frozen peas, washed
3 tablespoons fresh parsley, including stems and roots, washed and chopped
2 tablespoons fresh dill, washed and chopped
2 medium onions, moderately diced
1 handful wood ear mushrooms, previously soaked in water for 1 hour,
then washed and rinsed, wooden parts removed
1 teaspoon unrefined rock salt
4 tablespoons rice oil
2 tablespoons rice flour
1 cup spring water
2 teaspoons mixed herbs of your choice *(See also page 6.)*

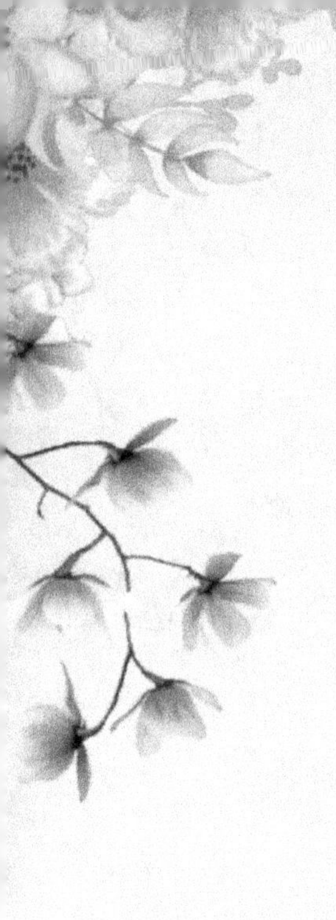
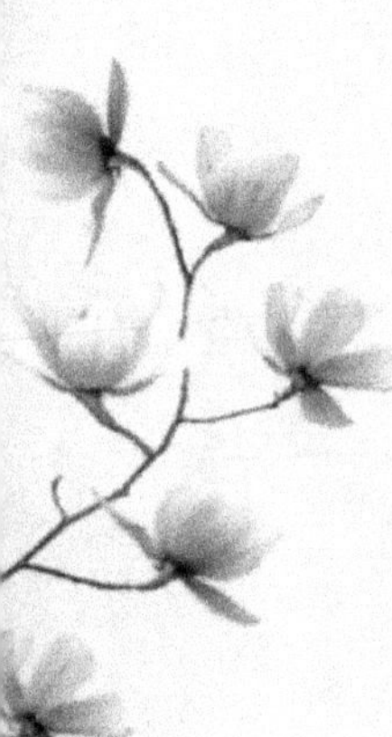

PREPARATION

1. Pour rice oil in a heavy skillet over medium heat.
2. Add carrots.
3. Stir for at least 1 minute.
4. Add pepper, mushrooms, peas, and beans.
5. Stir for at least 1 minute.
6. Add onion.
7. Stir gently.
8. Mix rice flour with vegetables.
9. Stir gently for a few seconds.
10. Add spring water.
11. Stir until creamy.
12. Add parsley and dill.
13. Stir for at least 1 minute.
14. Add seasonings and salt.
15. Stir for 30 seconds.
16. Remove skillet from heat.
17. Let it cool for 2 minutes.
18. Serve hot, warm, or at room temperature.

You Matter!

1. Take four gorgeous pictures of your culinary result.

2. Write down your impressions of the recipe.

a. Did you like it?

____

b. Was it difficult?

____

c. Did you find all the ingredients?

____

d. Did you make any changes to the recipe to better suit your dietary needs?

____

____

e. Will you cook it again?

____

f. Will you share it with your family and friends?

____

g. How did it make your body feel?

____

____

h. How were you feeling before cooking the recipe?

____

____

i. How were you feeling after eating the culinary result?

____

____

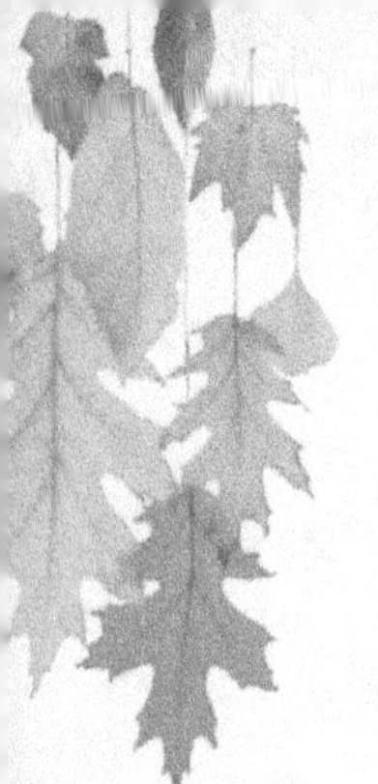

BAKED SQUASH

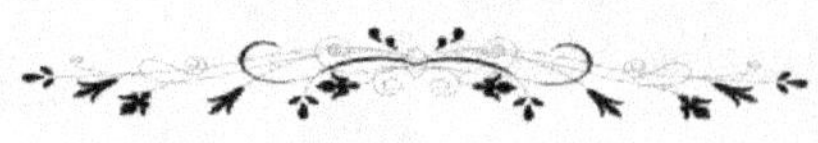

In case you didn't know, squash is botanically a fruit, although it has always been prepared and served as a vegetable.

Besides your culinary project 365, you can also enjoy the delicious, buttery texture of baked squash when anxiously waiting for some important results or news.

Type of Meal	Snack Dessert
Type of Dish	Vegetarian Non-Vegetarian
Preparation Time	Approximately 1 minute
Cooking Time	Approximately 1 hour
Servings	6
The AilamA® Cookbook advises You	Buttercup squashes are not as sweet as butternut ones, so you can enhance their taste by adding a healthy sweetener before or after baking them.

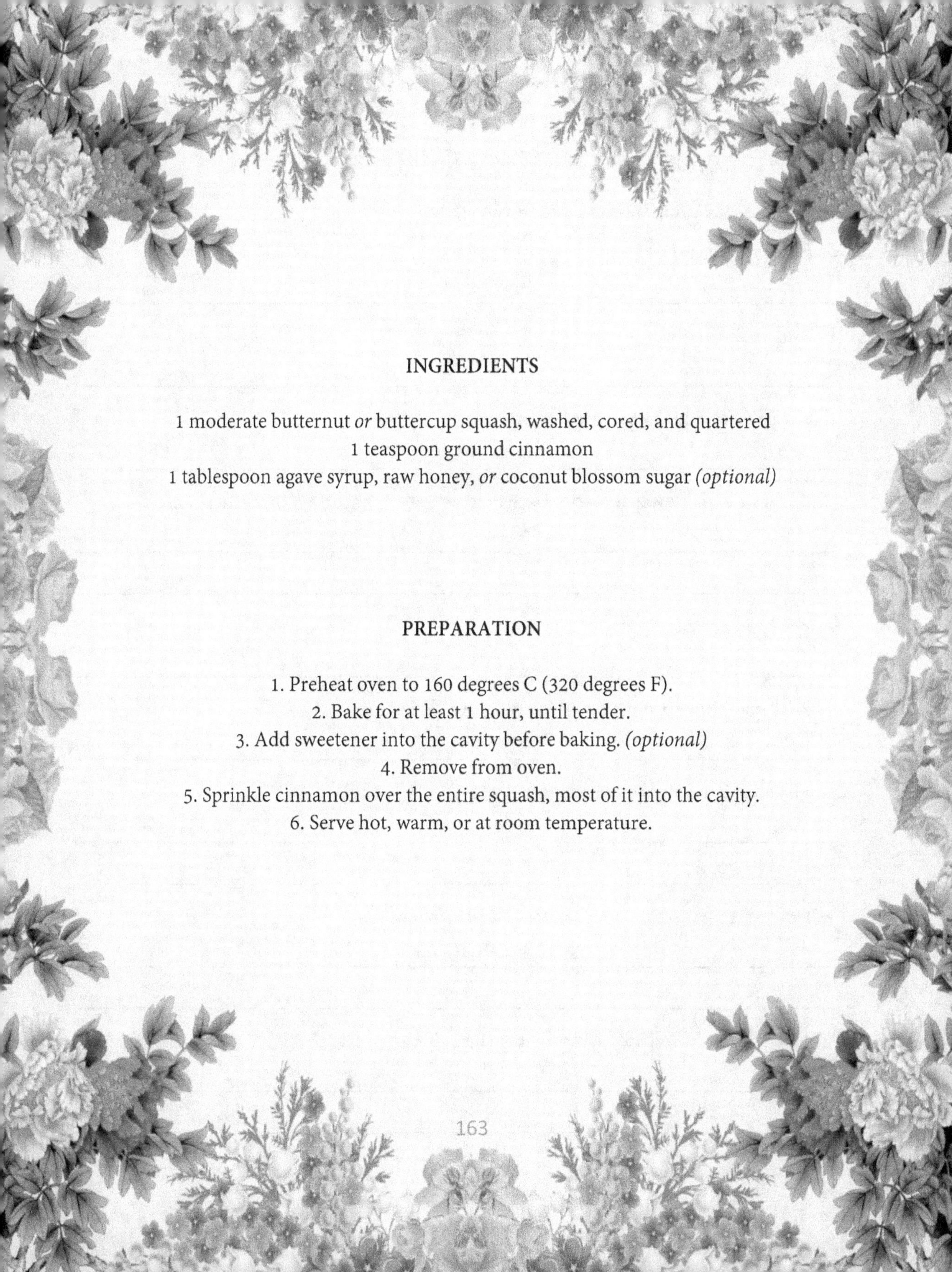

INGREDIENTS

1 moderate butternut *or* buttercup squash, washed, cored, and quartered
1 teaspoon ground cinnamon
1 tablespoon agave syrup, raw honey, *or* coconut blossom sugar *(optional)*

PREPARATION

1. Preheat oven to 160 degrees C (320 degrees F).
2. Bake for at least 1 hour, until tender.
3. Add sweetener into the cavity before baking. *(optional)*
4. Remove from oven.
5. Sprinkle cinnamon over the entire squash, most of it into the cavity.
6. Serve hot, warm, or at room temperature.

You Matter!

1. Take four gorgeous pictures of your culinary result.

2. Write down your impressions of the recipe.

a. Did you like it?

____

b. Was it difficult?

____

c. Did you find all the ingredients?

____

d. Did you make any changes to the recipe to better suit your dietary needs?

____

____

e. Will you cook it again?

____

f. Will you share it with your family and friends?

____

g. How did it make your body feel?

____

____

h. How were you feeling before cooking the recipe?

____

____

i. How were you feeling after eating the culinary result?

____

____

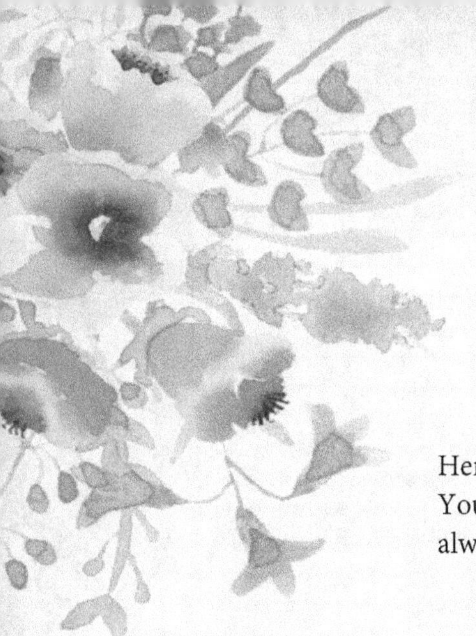

OLD SUSHI

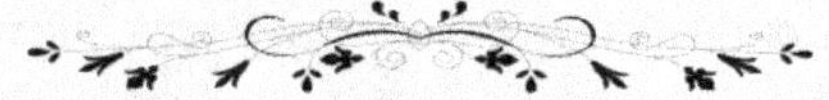

Here is a rapid recipe that is the closest to the classic sushi. You can also eat it in honor of your inflexible side, which always wants to maintain the status quo.

Type of Meal	Main Course
	Appetizer
	Snack
Type of Dish	Pesco-Ovo-Vegetarian
	Non-Vegetarian
Preparation Time	Approximately 10 minutes
	Approximately 20 minutes, boiling time
Cooking Time	Approximately 20 minutes
Servings	4
The AilamA® Cookbook advises You	Make sure you buy fresh, organic salmon, preferably the wild-caught type.

INGREDIENTS

2 sheets nori seaweed
1 cup sushi rice *or* basmati rice, previously boiled
1 large strip raw fresh salmon
2 long strips red pepper
2 strips cucumber
1 lemon, juiced
1 strip green salad
2 teaspoonfuls (germinated) sesame seeds
¼ cup parsley leaves *(optional)*
Pinch of unrefined rock salt
Pickled horseradish *or* grated ginger

PREPARATION

1. Put rice in a pot.
2. Cover it with spring water and add pinch of salt.
3. Bring rice to a boil.
4. Let it simmer until done.
5. Sprinkle it with sesame oil.
6. Mix well.
7. Let rice get cold.
8. Position nori seaweed on a bamboo sushi mat.
9. Spread a thin or thick layer of rice, as desired.
10. Dip salmon strip in sesame seeds on both sides.
11. Place it quite in the middle of nori sheet.
12. Add pepper, cucumber, salad, parsley.
13. Sprinkle with salt and lemon juice.
14. Roll to form sushi.
15. Slice with a sharp knife.
16. Serve with pickled horseradish or grated ginger on top.

You Matter!

1. Take four gorgeous pictures of your culinary result.

2. Write down your impressions of the recipe.

a. Did you like it?

____

b. Was it difficult?

____

c. Did you find all the ingredients?

____

d. Did you make any changes to the recipe to better suit your dietary needs?

____

____

e. Will you cook it again?

____

f. Will you share it with your family and friends?

____

g. How did it make your body feel?

____

____

h. How were you feeling before cooking the recipe?

____

____

i. How were you feeling after eating the culinary result?

____

____

BAKED QUINCE

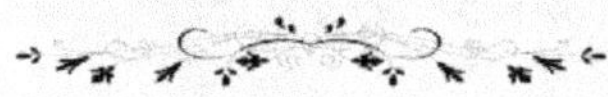

When baked, quinces are simply delicious, not to mention very
appealing to the eye thanks to their golden-brown look.
You can also eat baked quinces after you have wept buckets for
reasons best known to yourself.

Type of Meal	Snack
	Dessert
Type of Dish	Vegetarian
	Non-Vegetarian
Preparation Time	Approximately 1 minute
Cooking Time	Approximately 1 hour
Servings	8
The AilamA® Cookbook advises You	There is a big difference in taste between fresh and baked quinces. Keep that in mind if you've never baked them before.

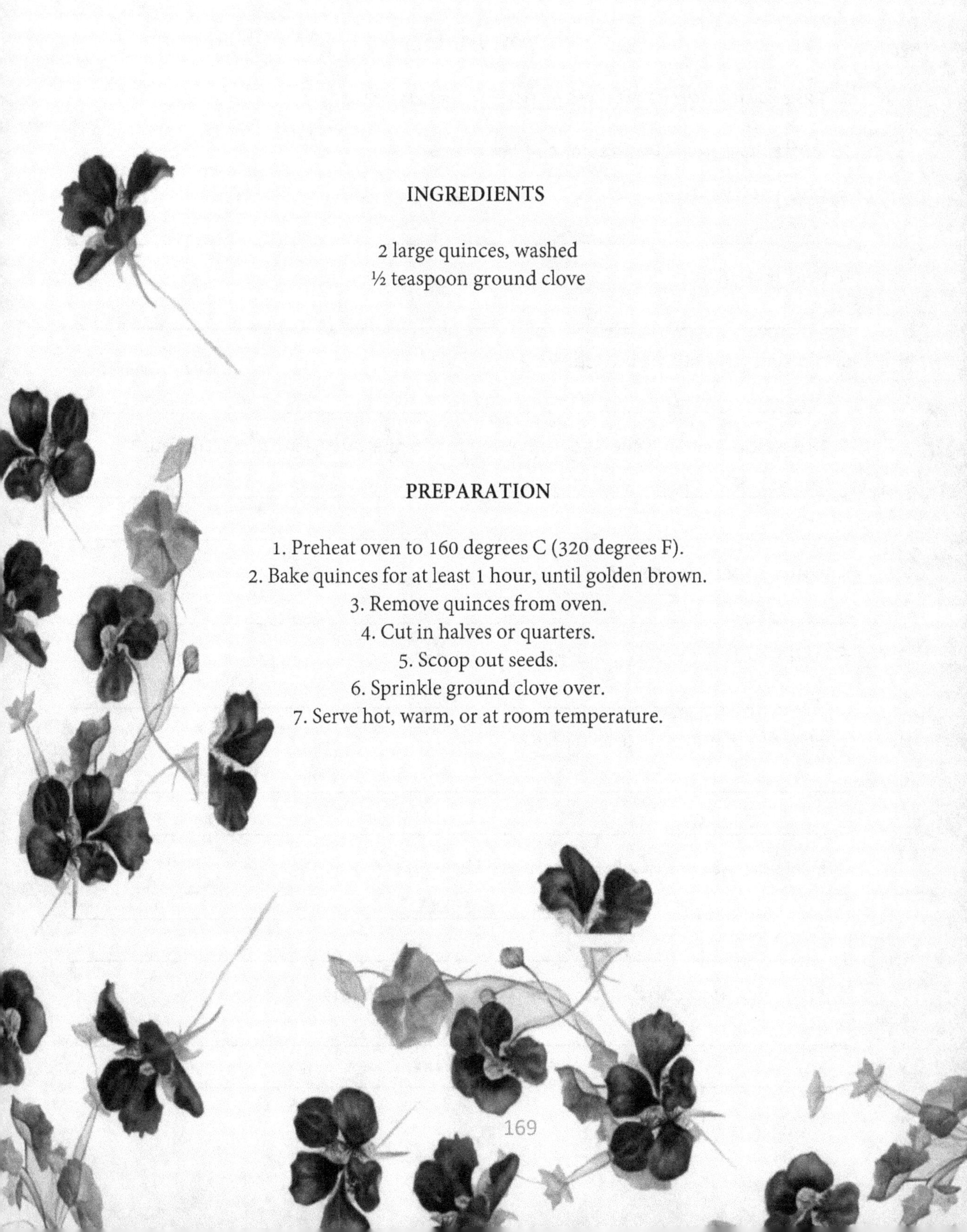

INGREDIENTS

2 large quinces, washed
½ teaspoon ground clove

PREPARATION

1. Preheat oven to 160 degrees C (320 degrees F).
2. Bake quinces for at least 1 hour, until golden brown.
3. Remove quinces from oven.
4. Cut in halves or quarters.
5. Scoop out seeds.
6. Sprinkle ground clove over.
7. Serve hot, warm, or at room temperature.

You Matter!

1. Take four gorgeous pictures of your culinary result.

2. Write down your impressions of the recipe.

a. Did you like it?

____

b. Was it difficult?

____

c. Did you find all the ingredients?

____

d. Did you make any changes to the recipe to better suit your dietary needs?

____

____

e. Will you cook it again?

____

f. Will you share it with your family and friends?

____

g. How did it make your body feel?

____

____

h. How were you feeling before cooking the recipe?

____

____

i. How were you feeling after eating the culinary result?

____

____

DINKEL FLATTIES

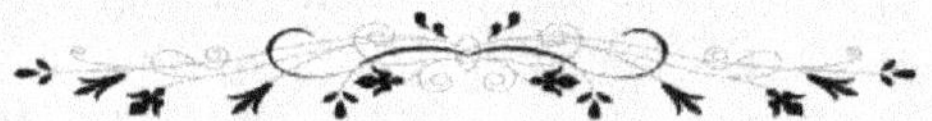

Spelt or dinkel is one of the healthiest species of wheat and therefore so is spelt flatbread. Whenever you feel exhausted, you can also eat this type of bread with something sweet, yet sugar-free, and your body will certainly thank you for your culinary choice.

Type of Meal	Snack Side Dish
Type of Dish	Vegetarian Non-Vegetarian
Preparation Time	Approximately 10 minutes, washing time Approximately 8 hours, soaking time
Cooking Time	Approximately 30 minutes
Servings	10 pieces
The AilamA® Cookbook advises You	If you don't want to make your own dinkel flour, you can buy a small bag of organic wholegrain spelt flour from any health food store or supermarket. Ceramic non-stick pans are much healthier and also better for the environment.

INGREDIENTS

5 tea cups *(or more)* organic spelt grains *(from any health food store)*
Pinch of natural salt
½ glass warm spring water *(or more)*
1 egg white *(optional)*

PREPARATION

SPELT FLOUR

1. Wash grains thoroughly until water comes out clear.
2. Soak grains in spring water overnight. *(optional)*
3. For optimal results, keep soaked grains in the refrigerator. *(optional)*
4. Rinse grains several times. *(optional)*
5. Put grains in oven at the lowest temperature setting.
6. Stir grains occasionally, until they become completely dry.
7. Let grains cool.
8. Grind grains into flour.

SPELT FLATBREAD

1. Put flour, salt, and egg white in a glass bowl.
2. Gradually add water while kneading the dough.
3. If dough is too sticky, add more flour.
4. If dough is too dry, add more water.
5. Knead dough until soft and not sticky.
6. Divide dough into small balls.
7. Flatten dough into thin discs with hands.
8. Heat a large ceramic pan.
9. Place pieces of flatbread in non-stick pan.
10. Cook for 1-2 minutes on one side.
11. Flip flatbread over.
12. Cook flatbread for 1-2 minutes on the other side.
13. Remove from heat.
14. Serve warm or cold with jam, preserve, vegetables, yoghurt, or cheese.

You Matter!

1. Take four gorgeous pictures of your culinary result.

2. Write down your impressions of the recipe.

a. Did you like it?

____

b. Was it difficult?

____

c. Did you find all the ingredients?

____

d. Did you make any changes to the recipe to better suit your dietary needs?

____

____

e. Will you cook it again?

____

f. Will you share it with your family and friends?

____

g. How did it make your body feel?

____

____

h. How were you feeling before cooking the recipe?

____

____

i. How were you feeling after eating the culinary result?

____

____

SWEET-SOUR COMFY

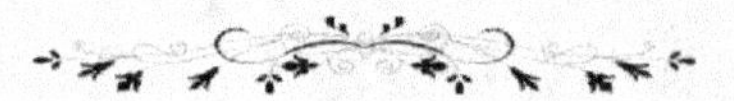

Are you feeling a bit down?
Here is a highly therapeutic cake to uplift your mood and balance your hormones, whenever necessary.
Make your thyroid your best friend with this tasty snack or dessert, which you can share with your family and friends.
Everyone deserves to be healthy!

Type of Meal	Snack
	Dessert
Type of Dish	Lacto-Ovo-Vegetarian
	Non-Vegetarian
Preparation Time	Approximately 10 minutes
Cooking Time	Approximately 25 minutes
Servings	16 pieces
The AilamA® Cookbook advises You	For best results, prepare the flour and the preserve at home. *(See also pages 143 and 171.)*

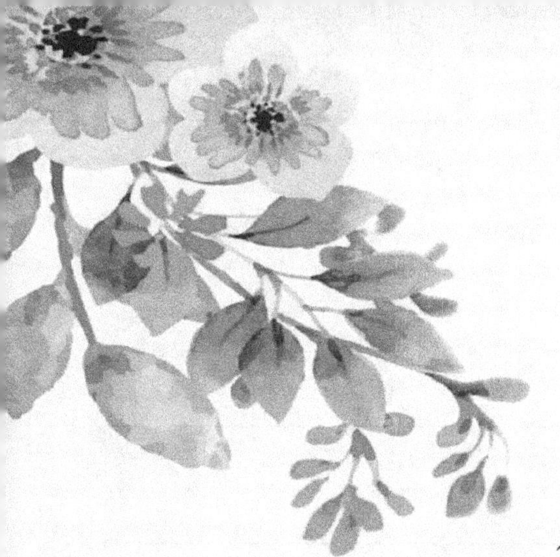

INGREDIENTS

2 egg whites
2 medium cups organic wholemeal spelt flour
1 small cup sugar-free sour cherry preserve *or* frozen sour cherries
1 glass *(or more)* coconut water from young, green coconut
Pinch of salt

PREPARATION

1. Preheat oven to 160 degrees C (320 degrees F).
2. Put flour, egg whites, salt, and coconut water in a glass baking dish.
3. Mix until well-blended and slightly runny.
4. Add preserve or frozen sour cherries.
5. Mix until well combined.
6. Bake for about 25 minutes or until golden brown.
7. Remove from oven.
8. Let cake cool.
9. Cut into small pieces.
10. Serve warm or at room temperature.

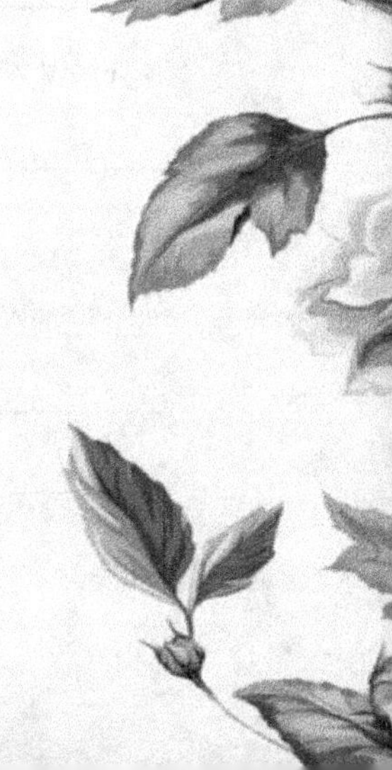

You Matter!

1. Take four gorgeous pictures of your culinary result.

2. Write down your impressions of the recipe.

a. Did you like it?

____

b. Was it difficult?

____

c. Did you find all the ingredients?

____

d. Did you make any changes to the recipe to better suit your dietary needs?

____

____

e. Will you cook it again?

____

f. Will you share it with your family and friends?

____

g. How did it make your body feel?

____

____

h. How were you feeling before cooking the recipe?

____

____

i. How were you feeling after eating the culinary result?

____

____

MASHED BLACK BEAN

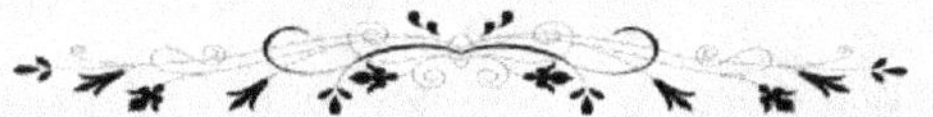

Here is yet another tasty, nutrient-dense dish for both meat-eaters and vegetarians. You can also have this healthy dish after you have been weighed up or criticized by a stranger.

Type of Meal	Main Course Snack
Type of Dish	Vegetarian Non-Vegetarian
Preparation Time	Approximately 5 minutes Approximately 8 hours, soaking time Approximately 15 minutes, baking time
Cooking Time	Approximately 2 hours
Servings	4
The AilamA® Cookbook advises You	Soak beans in cold water for at least 8 hours to improve their digestibility and reduce their hardness. Cook this type of protein with carrots and dried herbs to make it more digestible. Change water several times while you boil it. Always replace boiling water with warm to hot water.

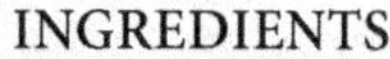

INGREDIENTS

1 egg
2 large cups black beans, previously soaked in spring water
4 large carrots, roughly cut
1 medium onion, previously baked
1 cup extra virgin olive oil
¼ teaspoon unrefined sea salt
4 teaspoons dried thyme
4 teaspoons dried basil
½ moderate lemon, juiced *(optional)*
1 tablespoon fresh parsley, washed and chopped
1½ teaspoons mixed herbs of your choice *(See also page 6.)*

PREPARATION

1. Put black beans in a pot.
2. Add spring water to cover them.
3. Boil them for 30 minutes with carrots, basil, and thyme.
4. Bring spring water to a boil in a separate pot.
5. Change beans' water 3 times, every 30 minutes.
6. Each time, add carrots, basil, and thyme.
7. Add 1 teaspoon mixed herbs in the final water.
8. Boil for 30 minutes or so, until beans become soft.
9. Meanwhile, bake onion for about 15 minutes.
10. Put boiled beans, oil, salt, egg, onion, and ½ mixed herbs in a blender.
11. Blend until smooth or coarsely consistent, as desired.
12. Add lemon juice until desired taste is obtained. *(optional)*
13. Transfer to a mixing bowl.
14. Add parsley.
15. Whisk it until smooth as desired.
16. Serve at room temperature, on slices of sweet red pepper or homemade bread.

You Matter!

1. Take four gorgeous pictures of your culinary result.

2. Write down your impressions of the recipe.

a. Did you like it?

____

b. Was it difficult?

____

c. Did you find all the ingredients?

____

d. Did you make any changes to the recipe to better suit your dietary needs?

____

____

e. Will you cook it again?

____

f. Will you share it with your family and friends?

____

g. How did it make your body feel?

____

____

h. How were you feeling before cooking the recipe?

____

____

i. How were you feeling after eating the culinary result?

____

____

CHICORY SWEET-EYED COOKIES

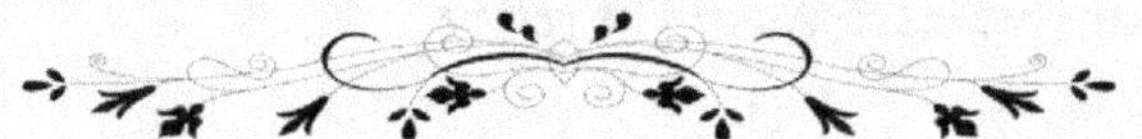

Here is a healthy cookie recipe that will keep you satiated for a long time. This dish also makes an excellent culinary companion when you go hiking with your family or friends.

Type of Meal	Snack
	Dessert
Type of Dish	Lacto-Ovo-Vegetarian
	Non-Vegetarian
Preparation Time	Approximately 10 minutes
	Approximately 30 minutes, refrigeration time
Cooking Time	Approximately 20 minutes
Servings	16 pieces
The AilamA® Cookbook advises You	Eating sweets right after a meal could create digestive disorders.

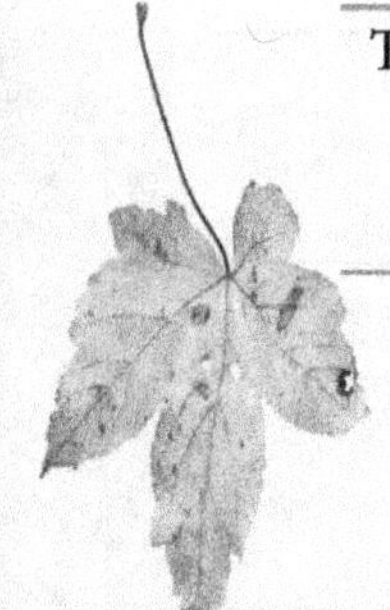

INGREDIENTS

1 large egg
1 small cup rice flour
½ pack butter
3 tablespoons coconut blossom sugar
½ small cup natural plum jam *or* preserve
2½ teaspoons chicory powder *or* instant chicory coffee powder
2 teaspoons (germinated) sesame seeds
2 teaspoons (germinated) walnuts, coarsely blended
2 teaspoons (germinated) almonds, coarsely blended
Cooking spray *(coconut oil)*
Pinch of salt

PREPARATION

1. Preheat oven to 160 degrees C (320 degrees F).
2. Put butter, sugar, and egg in a blender bowl.
3. Mix ingredients until light and fluffy.
4. Add flour, chicory powder, and salt.
5. Whisk until well combined.
6. Add walnuts and almonds.
7. Beat until combined.
8. Refrigerate batter for 30 minutes.
9. Roll dough into small balls.
10. Place on a baking sheet, lightly coated with cooking spray.
11. Add ¼ teaspoon plum jam on each ball.
12. Sprinkle with sesame seeds on top.
13. Bake for about 20 minutes, until golden brown.
14. Remove from oven.
15. Serve cold or at room temperature.

You Matter!

1. Take four gorgeous pictures of your culinary result.

2. Write down your impressions of the recipe.

a. Did you like it?

____

b. Was it difficult?

____

c. Did you find all the ingredients?

____

d. Did you make any changes to the recipe to better suit your dietary needs?

____

____

e. Will you cook it again?

____

f. Will you share it with your family and friends?

____

g. How did it make your body feel?

____

____

h. How were you feeling before cooking the recipe?

____

____

i. How were you feeling after eating the culinary result?

____

____

BROCCO WHITE DELIGHT

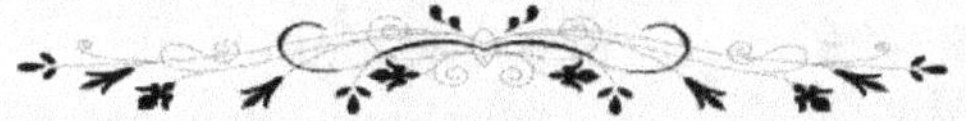

Here is a rapid broccoli stew for lunch or dinner. Enjoy!
You can also eat it after you have watched a horror movie or a broadcast that made you feel fearful and uneasy.

Type of Meal	Main Course
Type of Dish	Vegetarian Non-Vegetarian
Preparation Time	Approximately 10 minutes
Cooking Time	Approximately 5 minutes
Servings	4
The AilamA® Cookbook advises You	Broccoli is one of the many great detoxifiers that can help with weight loss. However, you should eat it together with seaweed, fish, or any other natural sources of iodine. Raw cruciferous vegetables, when consumed in large quantities, are bound to deplete iodine, thus making the thyroid gland sluggish and disrupting the whole hormonal system. A naturopath should also be consulted for extra information about goitrogens.

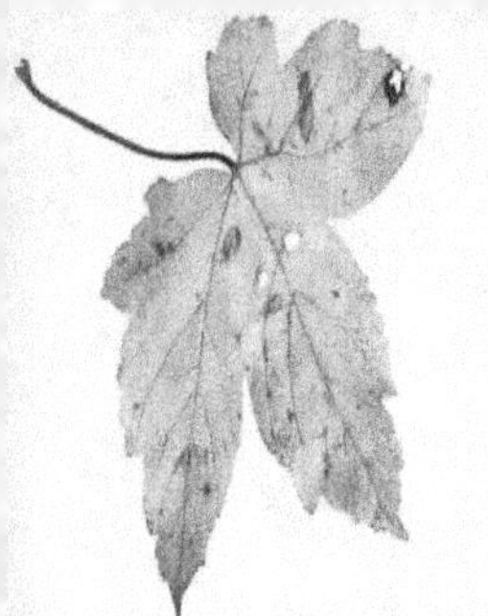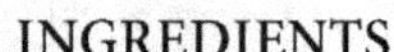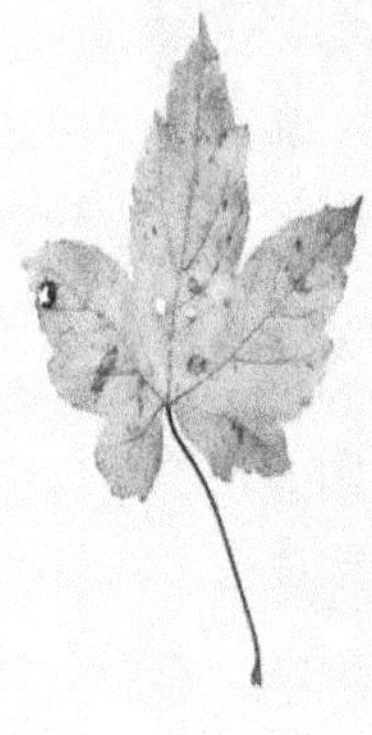

INGREDIENTS

1 large carrot, cut into moderate chunks
1 medium sweet red pepper, sliced lengthwise, then halved crosswise
4 handfuls fresh *or* frozen broccoli florets, washed and halved
2 tablespoons fresh parsley, including stems and roots, washed and chopped
2 medium onions moderately diced
3 cloves garlic, peeled and crushed
1 teaspoon unrefined sea salt
4 tablespoons rice oil
2 tablespoons rice flour
1 cup spring water
2 teaspoons mixed herbs of your choice *(See also page 6.)*

PREPARATION

1. Pour rice oil in a heavy skillet over medium heat.
2. Add broccoli.
3. Stir for at least 1 minute.
4. Add sweet red pepper and carrot.
5. Stir for at least 30 seconds.
6. Add onion and garlic.
7. Stir gently for 30 seconds.
8. Mix rice flour with vegetables.
9. Stir gently for 30 seconds.
10. Add spring water.
11. Stir until creamy.
12. Add parsley.
13. Stir for at least 30 seconds.
14. Add seasonings and salt.
15. Stir for 30 seconds.
16. Remove skillet from heat.
17. Let it cool for 1 minute.
18. Serve it hot or warm.

You Matter!

1. Take four gorgeous pictures of your culinary result.

2. Write down your impressions of the recipe.

a. Did you like it?

____

b. Was it difficult?

____

c. Did you find all the ingredients?

____

d. Did you make any changes to the recipe to better suit your dietary needs?

____

____

e. Will you cook it again?

____

f. Will you share it with your family and friends?

____

g. How did it make your body feel?

____

____

h. How were you feeling before cooking the recipe?

____

____

i. How were you feeling after eating the culinary result?

____

____

PLUM YUM-YUM

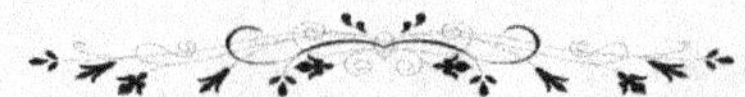

Did you know that jams, like preserves, could also be prepared entirely without sugar?
This healthy version of supermarket jams can also uplift your mood when you feel disappointed with yourself or when you are consumed with self-doubt and denial.

Type of Meal	Snack
	Dessert
Type of Dish	Vegetarian
	Non-Vegetarian
Preparation Time	Approximately 10 minutes
Cooking Time	Approximately 1 hour
Servings	4 small jars
The AilamA® Cookbook advises You	Being all natural, sugar-free jams should be kept in the refrigerator.
	For long-term preserving, you should keep the jars in the oven at low temperature for 1 hour.
	(See also page 143.)

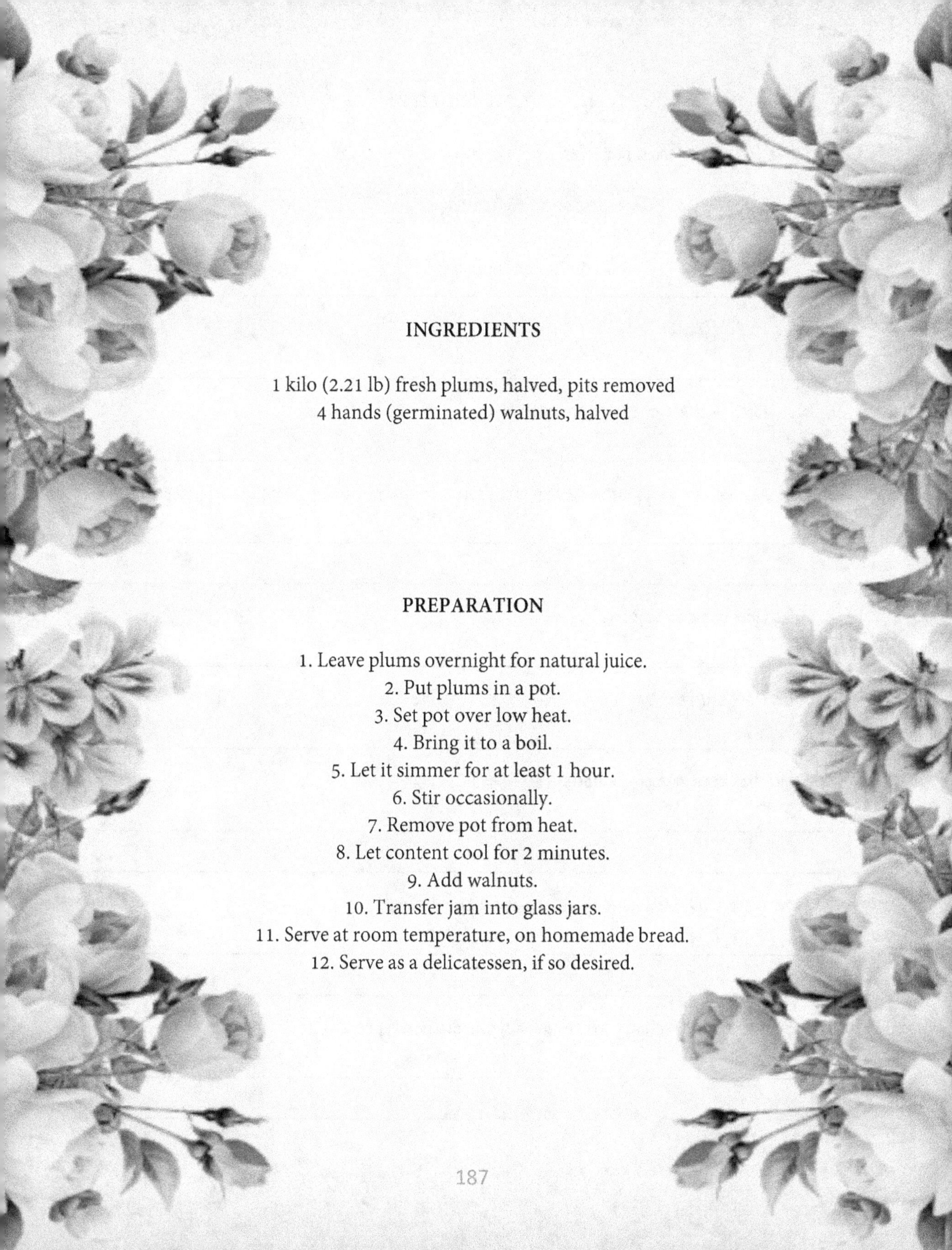

INGREDIENTS

1 kilo (2.21 lb) fresh plums, halved, pits removed
4 hands (germinated) walnuts, halved

PREPARATION

1. Leave plums overnight for natural juice.
2. Put plums in a pot.
3. Set pot over low heat.
4. Bring it to a boil.
5. Let it simmer for at least 1 hour.
6. Stir occasionally.
7. Remove pot from heat.
8. Let content cool for 2 minutes.
9. Add walnuts.
10. Transfer jam into glass jars.
11. Serve at room temperature, on homemade bread.
12. Serve as a delicatessen, if so desired.

You Matter!

1. Take four gorgeous pictures of your culinary result.

2. Write down your impressions of the recipe.

a. Did you like it?

____

b. Was it difficult?

____

c. Did you find all the ingredients?

____

d. Did you make any changes to the recipe to better suit your dietary needs?

____

____

e. Will you cook it again?

____

f. Will you share it with your family and friends?

____

g. How did it make your body feel?

____

____

h. How were you feeling before cooking the recipe?

____

____

i. How were you feeling after eating the culinary result?

____

____

BROIL & BAKE SALAD

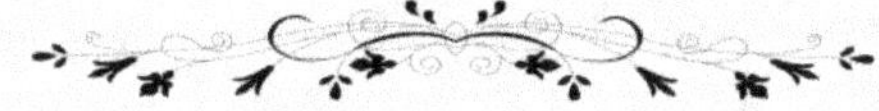

Broiled and baked vegetables should be a regular part of a
healthy eating plan, whether you are a vegetarian or not.
You can also have this salad whenever you are in low spirits.

Type of Meal	Snack
	Main Course
Type of Dish	Vegetarian
	Non-Vegetarian
Preparation Time	Approximately 10 minutes
Cooking Time	Approximately 15 minutes
Servings	4
The AilamA® Cookbook advises You	For this recipe, you can combine any type of vegetables you have on hand. Root vegetables require longer broiling or baking time.

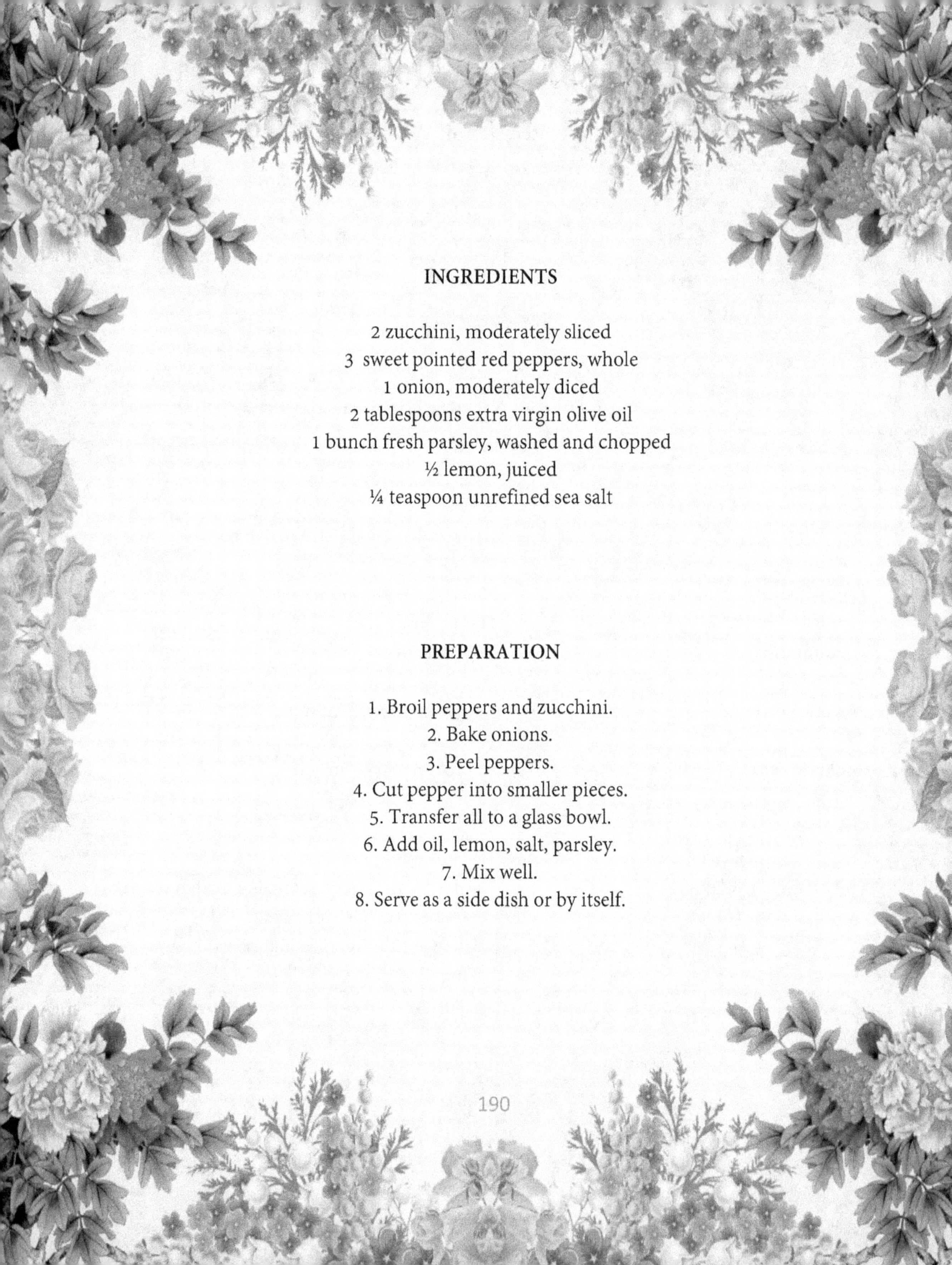

INGREDIENTS

2 zucchini, moderately sliced
3 sweet pointed red peppers, whole
1 onion, moderately diced
2 tablespoons extra virgin olive oil
1 bunch fresh parsley, washed and chopped
½ lemon, juiced
¼ teaspoon unrefined sea salt

PREPARATION

1. Broil peppers and zucchini.
2. Bake onions.
3. Peel peppers.
4. Cut pepper into smaller pieces.
5. Transfer all to a glass bowl.
6. Add oil, lemon, salt, parsley.
7. Mix well.
8. Serve as a side dish or by itself.

You Matter!

1. Take four gorgeous pictures of your culinary result.

2. Write down your impressions of the recipe.

a. Did you like it?

____

b. Was it difficult?

____

c. Did you find all the ingredients?

____

d. Did you make any changes to the recipe to better suit your dietary needs?

____

____

e. Will you cook it again?

____

f. Will you share it with your family and friends?

____

g. How did it make your body feel?

____

____

h. How were you feeling before cooking the recipe?

____

____

i. How were you feeling after eating the culinary result?

____

____

CARAMEL PUDDING

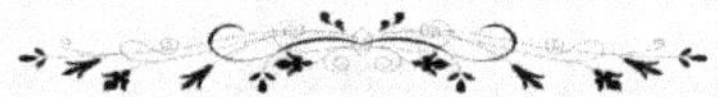

If you like caramelized sugar, here is a recipe you'll simply love, and so will your liver for that matter.

You can also binge on this sweet dish to honor the great power of your spirit to overcome difficulties.

Type of Meal	Snack Dessert
Type of Dish	Ovo-Vegetarian Non-Vegetarian
Preparation Time	Approximately 10 minutes
Cooking Time	Approximately 1½ hours
Servings	8
The AilamA® Cookbook advises You	The original recipe requires a large amount of white sugar and many whole eggs, which makes the result a real test for the liver. If you've tasted caramel pie or crème brûlée before, you'll see the fortunate difference as soon as you've tried this light and much healthier version.

INGREDIENTS

12 egg whites
4 tablespoons coconut blossom sugar
½ handful dried dates
6 tablespoons coconut milk diluted with 10 glasses spring water
Pinch of salt

PREPARATION

1. Preheat oven to 160 degrees C (320 degrees F).
2. Put a pot over a medium heat.
3. Add sugar.
4. Let it melt.
5. Spread it to brims.
6. Put pot aside to cool.
7. Put dates, egg whites, and salt in a blender.
8. Mix until light and fluffy.
9. Add diluted coconut milk.
10. Beat until well combined.
11. Pour runny content over caramel, no higher than sugar marks.
12. Put baking pot in a larger pot with water.
13. Bake for about 1½ hours or until jellified.
14. Remove from oven.
15. Let it cool.
16. Serve chilled or at room temperature.

You Matter!

1. Take four gorgeous pictures of your culinary result.

2. Write down your impressions of the recipe.

a. Did you like it?

____

b. Was it difficult?

____

c. Did you find all the ingredients?

____

d. Did you make any changes to the recipe to better suit your dietary needs?

____

____

e. Will you cook it again?

____

f. Will you share it with your family and friends?

____

g. How did it make your body feel?

____

____

h. How were you feeling before cooking the recipe?

____

____

i. How were you feeling after eating the culinary result?

____

____

CHEERFUL WOK

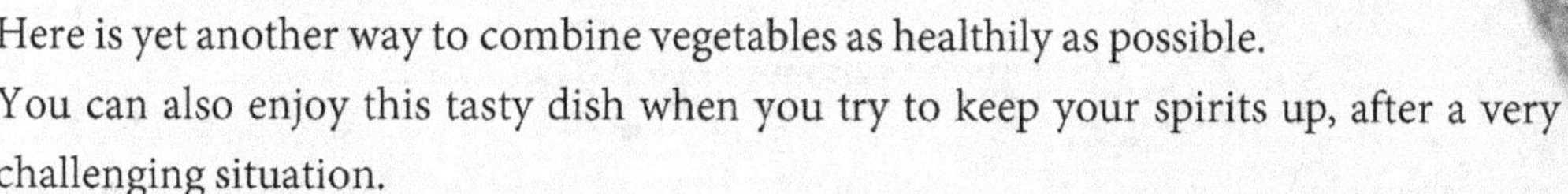

Here is yet another way to combine vegetables as healthily as possible.
You can also enjoy this tasty dish when you try to keep your spirits up, after a very
challenging situation.

Type of Meal	Main Course
Type of Dish	Vegetarian Non-Vegetarian
Preparation Time	Approximately 10 minutes Approximately 30 minutes, soaking time
Cooking Time	Approximately 15 minutes
Servings	4
The AilamA® Cookbook advises You	Always use long wooden or bamboo cooking utensils for stir-frying.

INGREDIENTS

1 large parsnip, sliced on the diagonal
½ medium celery root, cut into wedges
1 medium red pepper, sliced lengthwise, then halved
2 medium green zucchini, sliced lengthwise and cut into large chunks
1 bunch of lettuce, coarsely chopped with a wooden knife or torn into pieces by hand
2 medium onions, sliced in large rings
1 handful of seaweed, previously soaked in water for at least 30 minutes, then washed and rinsed
1 teaspoon unrefined rock salt
3 tablespoons rice oil
1 tablespoon pure sesame oil *(from roasted seeds)*
2 teaspoons mixed herbs of your choice *(See also page 6.)*
Meat (preferably turkey breast), prepared as desired and cut into bite-size pieces *(non-vegetarian dish)*

PREPARATION

1. Pour rice oil in a wok over medium-high heat.
2. Add parsnip, celery root, red pepper, and zucchini.
3. Stir-fry for at least 30 seconds.
4. Add onion.
5. Stir-fry until full rings separate into thin, hollow rings.
6. Add seaweed, lettuce, seasonings, and salt.
7. Stir-fry for at least 30 seconds.
8. Remove wok from heat.
9. Let it cool for 1 minute.
10. Add sesame oil.
11. Stir all ingredients one more time.
12. Add turkey breast. *(non-vegetarian dish)*
13. Stir one last time.
14. Serve hot, warm, or at room temperature.

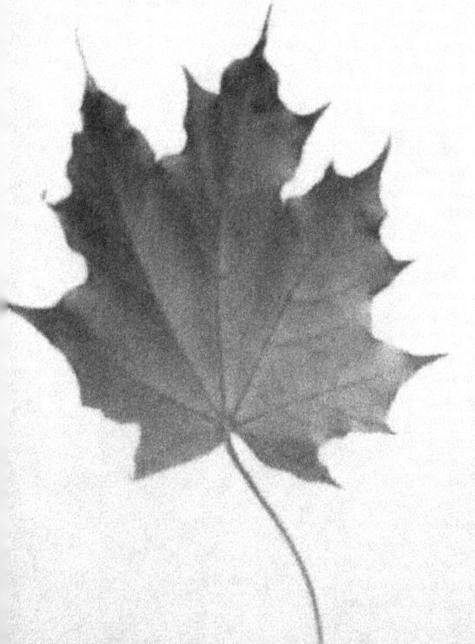

You Matter!

1. Take four gorgeous pictures of your culinary result.

2. Write down your impressions of the recipe.

a. Did you like it?

____

b. Was it difficult?

____

c. Did you find all the ingredients?

____

d. Did you make any changes to the recipe to better suit your dietary needs?

____

____

e. Will you cook it again?

____

f. Will you share it with your family and friends?

____

g. How did it make your body feel?

____

____

h. How were you feeling before cooking the recipe?

____

____

i. How were you feeling after eating the culinary result?

____

____

PICKLED CUCUMBERS

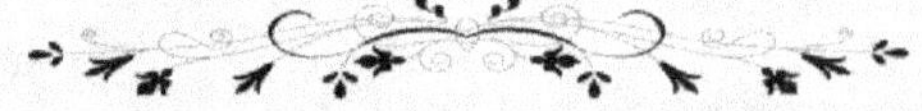

Here is the healthiest way to preserve cucumbers.
You can also eat pickled gherkins to honor the gut-brain axis.
Keep your gut healthy to keep your wholeness healthy !

Type of Meal	Main Course
	Dinner
Type of Dish	Vegetarian
	Non-Vegetarian
Preparation Time	Approximately 30 minutes
Cooking Time	Approximately 20 minutes, 3 days in a row
Servings	2 jars
The AilamA® Cookbook advises You	You can replace dried thyme and cumin seeds with dill and garlic, if you like this traditional combination better. But keep in mind that dried thyme and cumin are considered much better digestive aids. Gherkins should not move in the glass jar or start floating when you add the hot brine.
	It is better to prepare more brine than you need rather than being short of brine, hence the large quantity of spring water for 1 kilo (2.21 lbs) of gherkins.

INGREDIENTS

1 kilo (2.21 lbs) gherkin cucumbers
1½ liter (51 fl oz) spring water
1 tablespoon unrefined rock salt
1 tablespoon dried thyme
1 tablespoon cumin seeds

PREPARATION

1. Bring water to a boil.
2. Put salt in water.
3. Let salted water simmer for 2 minutes.
4. Wash gherkins in cold water.
5. Place gherkins in 2 glass jars.
6. Remove brine from heat.
7. Pour hot brine over gherkins.
8. Place perfect-sized lids on top of jars, preferably covered by a screw-on ring.
9. Do not tighten lids yet.
10. Store jars in a cool, dark place.
11. After 24 hours, empty brine from jars.
12. Bring brine to a boil.
13. Let brine simmer for 1 minute.
14. Wash cucumbers and jars with cold water.
15. Place cucumbers back into jars.
16. Pour hot brine over cucumbers.
17. Place lids on top of jars without tightening them.
18. Store jars in a cool, dark place.
19. After another 24 hours, empty brine from jars.
20. Bring brine to a boil.
21. Let brine simmer for 1 minute.
22. Wash cucumbers and jars with cold water.
23. Place cucumbers back into jars.
24. Put cumin and dried thyme in jars, ½ tablespoon of each in each jar.
25. Pour hot brine over cucumbers.
26. Seal jars with lids.
27. Store jars in a cool, dark place.
28. Serve with meat, salads, or grain dishes.

You Matter!

1. Take four gorgeous pictures of your culinary result.

2. Write down your impressions of the recipe.

a. Did you like it?

____

b. Was it difficult?

____

c. Did you find all the ingredients?

____

d. Did you make any changes to the recipe to better suit your dietary needs?

____

____

e. Will you cook it again?

____

f. Will you share it with your family and friends?

____

g. How did it make your body feel?

____

____

h. How were you feeling before cooking the recipe?

____

____

i. How were you feeling after eating the culinary result?

____

____

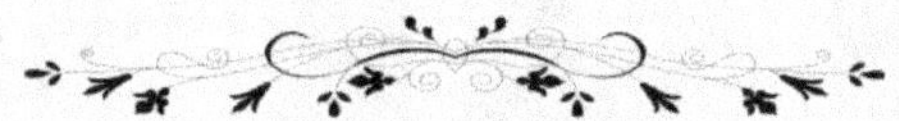

STIR FRIED EGGPLANTS

Here is yet another wok recipe beneficial to your health.

You can also eat this food to celebrate the harmony, creativity, and health of your physicality.

Type of Meal	Main Course
Type of Dish	Vegetarian Non-Vegetarian
Preparation Time	Approximately 10 minutes
Cooking Time	Approximately 10 minutes
Servings	4
The AilamA® Cookbook advises You	Eggplant chunks absorb a lot of oil. If you feel that 5 tablespoons aren't enough, just add some more so that the wok pot will remain slightly oily at the end of the cooking time. When done, eggplants should have a light brown colour and a mushroomy texture.

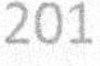

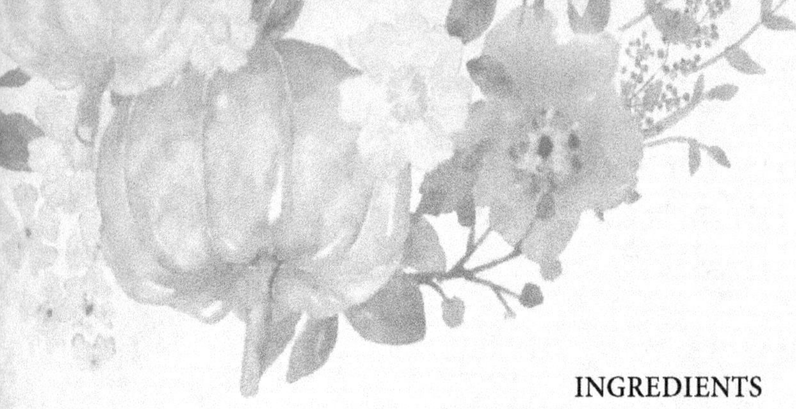

INGREDIENTS

3 large eggplants, cut lengthwise then moderately sliced
2 medium sweet red peppers, sliced lengthwise then halved
5 tablespoons fresh parsley, including stems and roots, washed and chopped
2 medium onions, sliced in full rings
2 celery stalks, moderately cut
2 tablespoons celery leaves, washed and chopped
1 teaspoon unrefined sea salt
6 cloves garlic, minced
5 tablespoons coconut oil
2 teaspoons mixed herbs of your choice *(See also page 6.)*
Meat (preferably beef or venison), prepared as desired, cut into bite-size pieces *(non-vegetarian dish)*

PREPARATION

1. Pour coconut oil in a wok over medium-high heat.
2. Add eggplants.
3. Stir-fry for at least 1 minute.
4. Add red peppers, onion, garlic, celery stalks and leaves.
5. Stir-fry for at least 30 seconds.
6. Add parsley, seasonings, and salt.
7. Stir-fry for at least 10 seconds.
8. Remove wok from heat.
9. Let it cool for 30 seconds.
10. Add meat. *(non-vegetarian dish)*
13. Stir one last time.
14. Serve hot or warm.

You Matter!

1. Take four gorgeous pictures of your culinary result.

2. Write down your impressions of the recipe.

a. Did you like it?

____

b. Was it difficult?

____

c. Did you find all the ingredients?

____

d. Did you make any changes to the recipe to better suit your dietary needs?

____

____

e. Will you cook it again?

____

f. Will you share it with your family and friends?

____

g. How did it make your body feel?

____

____

h. How were you feeling before cooking the recipe?

____

____

i. How were you feeling after eating the culinary result?

____

____

CINNAMON SPICE SWEET

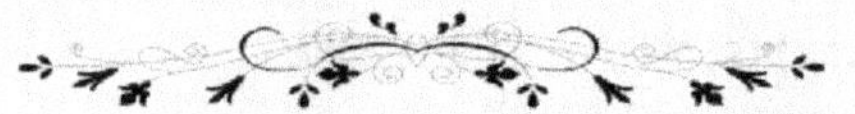

Here is another dish prepared with healthy ingredients to satisfy your craving for sweets … and love.

Type of Meal	Snack
	Dessert
Type of Dish	Lacto-Ovo-Vegetarian
	Non-Vegetarian
Preparation Time	Approximately 10 minutes
	Approximately 30 minutes, refrigeration time
Cooking Time	Approximately 30 minutes
Servings	16 pieces
The AilamA® Cookbook advises You	Feel free to experiment with this recipe.

INGREDIENTS

1 large egg
½ pack butter
1 cup rice flour
3 tablespoons coconut blossom sugar
½ small cup natural plum jam
4 tablespoons (germinated) almonds, coarsely ground
2 tablespoons (germinated) sesame seeds
3 teaspoons ground cinnamon
1 teaspoon ground clove
Cooking spray *(coconut oil)*
Pinch of salt

PREPARATION

1.Preheat oven to 160 degrees C (320 degrees F).
2. Put butter, sugar, and egg in a blender.
3. Mix ingredients until light and fluffy.
4. Whisk flour, salt, cinnamon, clove, and almonds in a separate glass bowl.
5. Add content to fluffy batter.
6. Whisk until well combined.
7. Refrigerate batter for 30 minutes.
8. Spread batter on a baking sheet, lightly coated with cooking spray.
9. Spread plum jam on it.
10. Sprinkle with sesame seeds all over.
11. Bake for about 20 minutes.
12. Remove from oven.
13. Cut when cold.
14. Serve cold or at room temperature.

You Matter!

1. Take four gorgeous pictures of your culinary result.

2. Write down your impressions of the recipe.

a. Did you like it?

____

b. Was it difficult?

____

c. Did you find all the ingredients?

____

d. Did you make any changes to the recipe to better suit your dietary needs?

____

____

e. Will you cook it again?

____

f. Will you share it with your family and friends?

____

g. How did it make your body feel?

____

____

h. How were you feeling before cooking the recipe?

____

____

i. How were you feeling after eating the culinary result?

____

____

SWEET POTATO SALAD

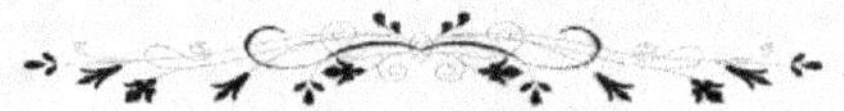

It's salty-sweet with a touch of crunchiness. You can have this nutritious salad for breakfast or dinner, you choose. Perhaps lunch?
You can also add it to your meals whenever you want to celebrate the joys of your romantic life.

Type of Meal	Snack
	Main Course
Type of Dish	Vegetarian
	Non-Vegetarian
Preparation Time	Approximately 10 minutes
	Approximately 1 hour, boiling or baking time
Cooking Time	Approximately 1 hour
Servings	4
The AilamA® Cookbook advises You	Natural olives have a brownish colour. If they are too salty, soak them in water for at least 30 minutes prior to using them.

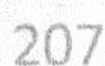

INGREDIENTS

6 large sweet potatoes, previously boiled/baked with herbs and salt
1 bunch parsley, washed and chopped
2 celery stalks, thinly sliced
2 medium sweet red peppers, sliced lengthwise, then halved crosswise
2 tablespoons unrefined sesame oil
1½ cups kalamata *or* green olives
1 onion, diced small
½ teaspoon unrefined rock salt
¼ teaspoon mixed herbs of your choice *(See also page 6.)*

PREPARATION

1. Cut potatoes in moderate chunks.
2. Put them into a glass bowl.
3. Add red pepper, celery, parsley, onion, olives, salt, herbs, and sesame oil.
4. Mix well.
5. Serve warm or at room temperature.

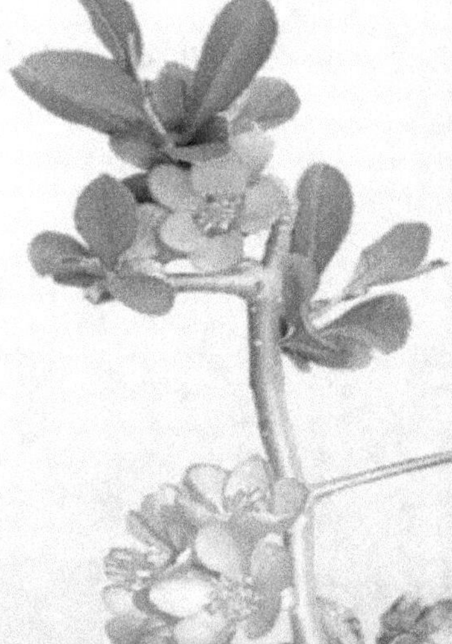

You Matter!

1. Take four gorgeous pictures of your culinary result.

2. Write down your impressions of the recipe.

a. Did you like it?

____

b. Was it difficult?

____

c. Did you find all the ingredients?

____

d. Did you make any changes to the recipe to better suit your dietary needs?

____

____

e. Will you cook it again?

____

f. Will you share it with your family and friends?

____

g. How did it make your body feel?

____

____

h. How were you feeling before cooking the recipe?

____

____

i. How were you feeling after eating the culinary result?

____

____

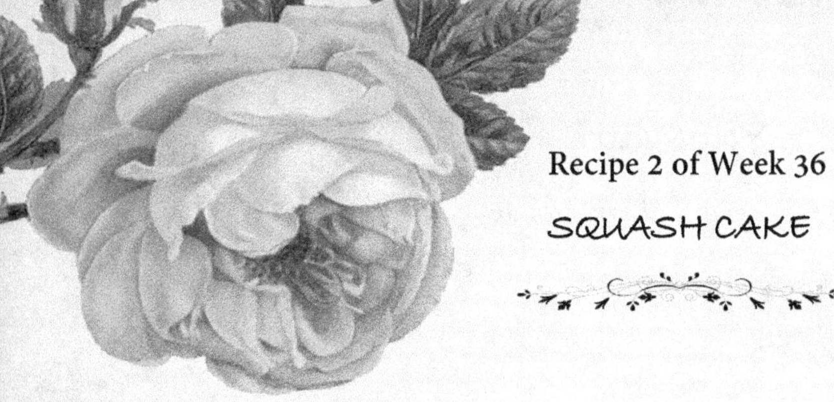

SQUASH CAKE

Here is yet another recipe that proves how healthy sweet dishes can actually be if prepared the right way.

This cake can also become your true friend when you are preoccupied and/or on the go all day.

Type of Meal	Snack Dessert
Type of Dish	Lacto-Ovo-Vegetarian Non-Vegetarian
Preparation Time	Approximately 10 minutes Approximately 30 minutes, refrigeration time
Cooking Time	Approximately 30 minutes
Servings	16 pieces
The AilamA® Cookbook advises You	Butternut squashes are quite sweet, so it's entirely up to you how much sweetener you will add to this recipe.

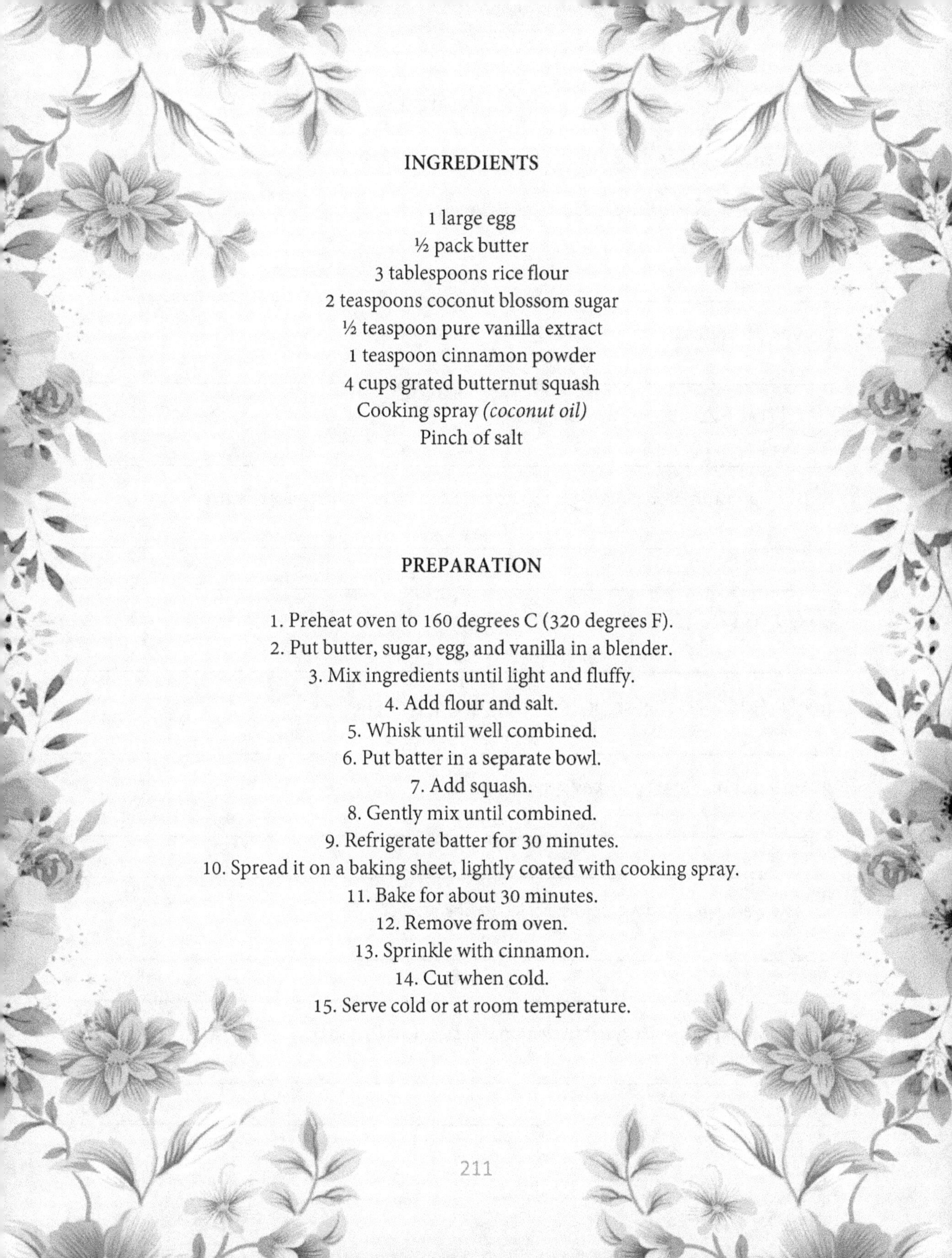

INGREDIENTS

1 large egg
½ pack butter
3 tablespoons rice flour
2 teaspoons coconut blossom sugar
½ teaspoon pure vanilla extract
1 teaspoon cinnamon powder
4 cups grated butternut squash
Cooking spray *(coconut oil)*
Pinch of salt

PREPARATION

1. Preheat oven to 160 degrees C (320 degrees F).
2. Put butter, sugar, egg, and vanilla in a blender.
3. Mix ingredients until light and fluffy.
4. Add flour and salt.
5. Whisk until well combined.
6. Put batter in a separate bowl.
7. Add squash.
8. Gently mix until combined.
9. Refrigerate batter for 30 minutes.
10. Spread it on a baking sheet, lightly coated with cooking spray.
11. Bake for about 30 minutes.
12. Remove from oven.
13. Sprinkle with cinnamon.
14. Cut when cold.
15. Serve cold or at room temperature.

You Matter!

1. Take four gorgeous pictures of your culinary result.

2. Write down your impressions of the recipe.

a. Did you like it?

____

b. Was it difficult?

____

c. Did you find all the ingredients?

____

d. Did you make any changes to the recipe to better suit your dietary needs?

____

____

e. Will you cook it again?

____

f. Will you share it with your family and friends?

____

g. How did it make your body feel?

____

____

h. How were you feeling before cooking the recipe?

____

____

i. How were you feeling after eating the culinary result?

____

____

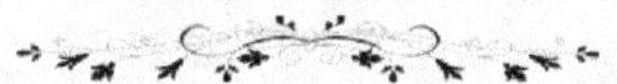

Here is the recipe of yet another delicious wok, prepared with one of the healthiest cruciferous vegetables.
You can also have this wok dish when you feel helpless because there's nothing you can do to make a situation better.

Type of Meal	Main Course
Type of Dish	Vegetarian Non-Vegetarian
Preparation Time	Approximately 10 minutes Approximately 15 minutes, boiling time
Cooking Time	Approximately 5 minutes
Servings	4
The AilamA® Cookbook advises You	Like broccoli, cabbage can affect your thyroid, especially when eaten raw. Always cook your cruciferous vegetables, if you suffer from hypothyroidism or other hormonal dysfunctions. (*See also page 183.*)

INGREDIENTS

2 medium sweet red peppers, sliced lengthwise, then halved crosswise
1 handful green beans, previously boiled, halved
1 cup frozen peas, washed
3 tablespoons fresh parsley, including stems and roots, washed and chopped
2 medium onions, thinly sliced crosswise
¼ moderate white cabbage, cut into large pieces
3 nectarines, stone removed, cut into moderate pieces
½ teaspoon unrefined sea salt
4 tablespoons rice oil
2 teaspoons mixed herbs of your choice *(See also page 6.)*
Meat (preferably chicken breast), prepared as desired, cut into bite-size pieces *(non-vegetarian dish)*

PREPARATION

1. Pour rice oil in a wok over high heat.
2. Add cabbage.
3. Stir-fry for at least 3 minutes.
4. Add pepper, peas, beans, onion, and nectarines.
5. Stir-fry for at least 30 seconds.
6. Add seasonings and salt.
7. Stir-fry for at least 30 seconds.
8. Remove wok from heat.
9. Add meat. *(non-vegetarian dish)*
10. Stir one last time.
11. Let it cool for 30 seconds.
12. Serve it hot, warm, or at room temperature.

You Matter!

1. Take four gorgeous pictures of your culinary result.

2. Write down your impressions of the recipe.

a. Did you like it?

____

b. Was it difficult?

____

c. Did you find all the ingredients?

____

d. Did you make any changes to the recipe to better suit your dietary needs?

____

____

e. Will you cook it again?

____

f. Will you share it with your family and friends?

____

g. How did it make your body feel?

____

____

h. How were you feeling before cooking the recipe?

____

____

i. How were you feeling after eating the culinary result?

____

____

Have you ever thought you can make fermented cheese from homemade kefir? The result is not only healthy, but also highly therapeutic. The only downside is that, from 1 liter of kefir, you'll get only a small amount of this tasty sour cheese, along with a large quantity of fermented whey.

You can also eat this cheese as a reminder of the creative person that you are, who turns downsides into upsides.

Type of Meal	Snack
	Appetizer
Type of Dish	Lacto-Vegetarian
	Non-Vegetarian
Preparation Time	1 day, fermentation time for kefir
Cooking Time	Approximately 3 minutes
Servings	8
The AilamA® Cookbook advises You	You can drink the remaining whey or use it for making pancakes. Either way, you'll get double benefits from its fermentation. You can also add dried herbs like dill, cumin, thyme, or turmeric, for extra flavor and nice color.
	(See also pages 25 and 38.)

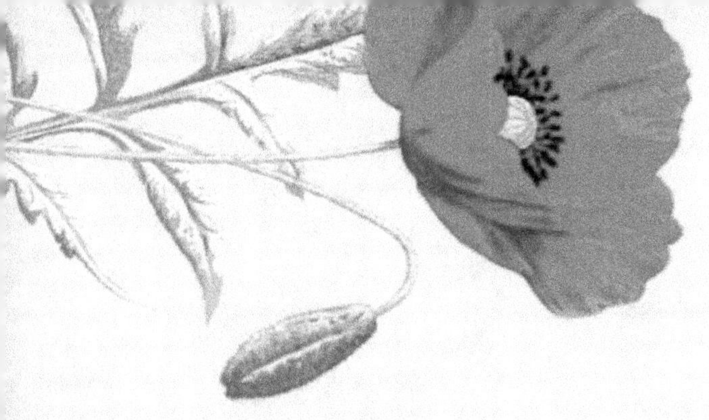
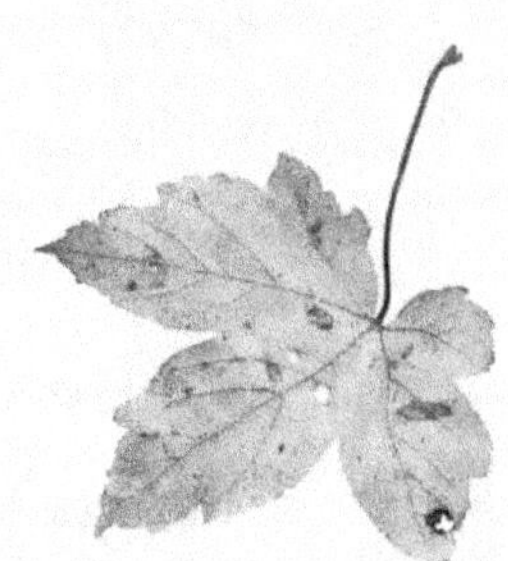

INGREDIENTS

1 liter (~35 fl oz) homemade kefir
1 tablespoon unrefined rock salt

PREPARATION

1. Add salt to kefir.
2. Heat kefir at low temperature.
3. Let kefir warm until small curds separate from whey.
4. Don't stir kefir.
5. Let curdled kefir cool.
6. Leave curdled kefir in a strain, until no more fermented whey comes out.
7. Serve cold, chilled, or at room temperature.

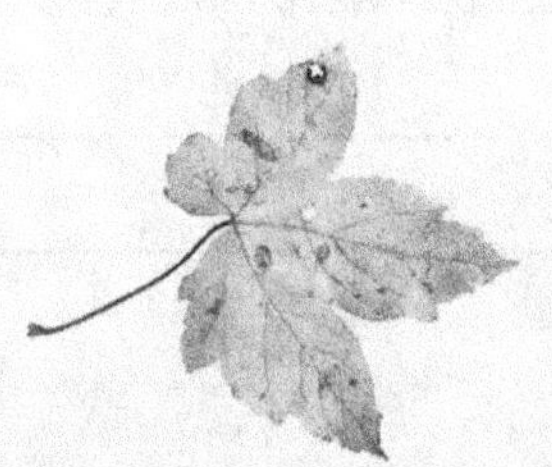

You Matter!

1. Take four gorgeous pictures of your culinary result.

2. Write down your impressions of the recipe.

a. Did you like it?

____

b. Was it difficult?

____

c. Did you find all the ingredients?

____

d. Did you make any changes to the recipe to better suit your dietary needs?

____

____

e. Will you cook it again?

____

f. Will you share it with your family and friends?

____

g. How did it make your body feel?

____

____

h. How were you feeling before cooking the recipe?

____

____

i. How were you feeling after eating the culinary result?

____

____

K-SUSHI

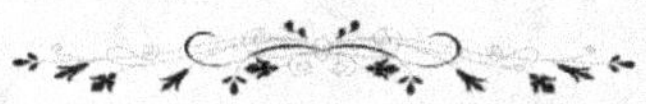

Here is yet another sushi dish for you and your family, prepared with simple and healthy ingredients.

You can also have it to celebrate your unstinting devotion to a noble cause.

Type of Meal	Main Course
	Appetizer
	Snack
Type of Dish	Lacto-Ovo-Vegetarian
	Non-Vegetarian
Preparation Time	Approximately 10 minutes
	Approximately 20 minutes, boiling time
Cooking Time	Approximately 20 minutes
Servings	4
The AilamA® Cookbook advises You	Kefir cheese is packed with probiotics, which makes this sushi recipe quite unique.

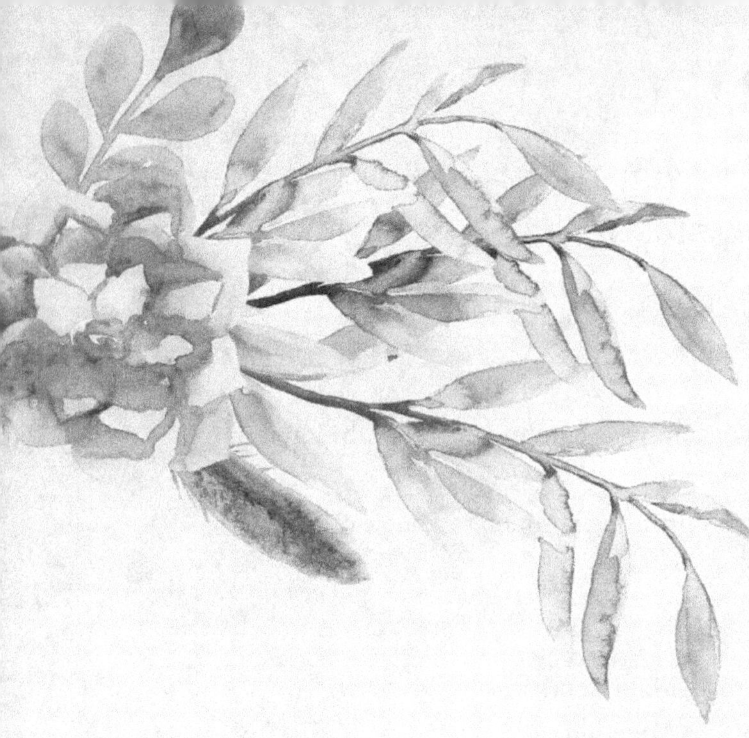

INGREDIENTS

2 sheets nori seaweed
2 egg whites
Cooking spray *(coconut oil)*
¼ cup chopped fresh parsley
3 tablespoons kefir cheese
2 long strips sweet pointed red pepper
Pinch of salt
Pickled horseradish, grated *(optional)*
Fresh ginger, grated *(optional)*

PREPARATION

1. Beat egg whites, kefir cheese, and parsley in a glass bowl.
9. Add pinch of salt.
10. Spray pan with coconut oil.
11. Make egg white omelet.
12. Let omelet get cold.
13. Position nori seaweed on a sushi mat.
14. Spread cold omelet on nori.
15. Add red pepper.
16. Sprinkle with salt, if needed.
17. Roll to form sushi.
18. Slice it with a sharp knife.
19. Serve with grated pickled horseradish or fresh ginger on top, if so desired.

You Matter!

1. Take four gorgeous pictures of your culinary result.

2. Write down your impressions of the recipe.

a. Did you like it?

____

b. Was it difficult?

____

c. Did you find all the ingredients?

____

d. Did you make any changes to the recipe to better suit your dietary needs?

____

____

e. Will you cook it again?

____

f. Will you share it with your family and friends?

____

g. How did it make your body feel?

____

____

h. How were you feeling before cooking the recipe?

____

____

i. How were you feeling after eating the culinary result?

____

____

WOK DELIGHT

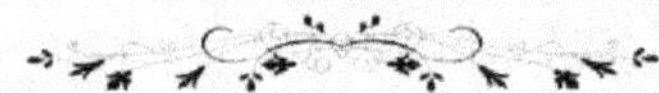

Here is yet another healthy wok recipe for you and your family. It can also accompany your reflection on the implications of a certain decision you have made recently.

Type of Meal	Main Course
Type of Dish	Vegetarian Non-Vegetarian
Preparation Time	Approximately 10 minutes Approximately 30 minutes, boiling time Approximately 1 hour, soaking time
Cooking Time	Approximately 15 minutes
Servings	4
The AilamA® Cookbook advises You	Wash bamboo shoots thoroughly in cold water, especially if they have been preserved in citric acid. Then let them soak in cold water for at least 6 hours and change their water periodically. Take a medium bamboo shoot and boil it with seasonings for at least 30 minutes before using it in your woks.

INGREDIENTS

1 large parsnip, cut into large chunks
½ medium bamboo shoots, thinly sliced
¼ buttercup squash, cut into large chunks
1 medium sweet pointed red pepper, sliced lengthwise then halved
2 medium green zucchini, sliced lengthwise and cut into large chunks
1 medium quince, cut in large chunks
5 tablespoons fresh parsley, including stems and roots, washed and chopped
2 medium onions, sliced in full rings
2 handfuls of wood ear mushrooms, previously soaked in water for at least 1 hour,
then washed and rinsed, wooden parts removed
1 teaspoon unrefined rock salt
3 tablespoons rice oil
1 tablespoon pure sesame oil *(from roasted seeds)*
2 teaspoons mixed herbs of your choice *(See also page 6.)*
Meat (preferably chicken breast),
prepared as desired and cut into bite-size pieces *(non-vegetarian dish)*

PREPARATION

1. Pour rice oil in a wok over medium-high heat.
2. Add parsnip, buttercup squash, pepper, zucchini, bamboo shoots, mushrooms, and quince.
3. Stir-fry for at least 2 minutes.
4. Add onion.
5. Stir-fry until full rings separate into thin hollow rings.
6. Add parsley, seasonings, and salt.
7. Stir-fry for 20 seconds.
8. Remove wok from heat.
9. Let it cool for 30 seconds.
10. Add sesame oil.
11. Add chicken breast. *(non-vegetarian dish)*
12. Stir all ingredients one more time.
13. Serve hot, warm, or at room temperature.

You Matter!

1. Take four gorgeous pictures of your culinary result.

2. Write down your impressions of the recipe.

a. Did you like it?

____

b. Was it difficult?

____

c. Did you find all the ingredients?

____

d. Did you make any changes to the recipe to better suit your dietary needs?

____

____

e. Will you cook it again?

____

f. Will you share it with your family and friends?

____

g. How did it make your body feel?

____

____

h. How were you feeling before cooking the recipe?

____

____

i. How were you feeling after eating the culinary result?

____

____

RASPBERRY CAKE

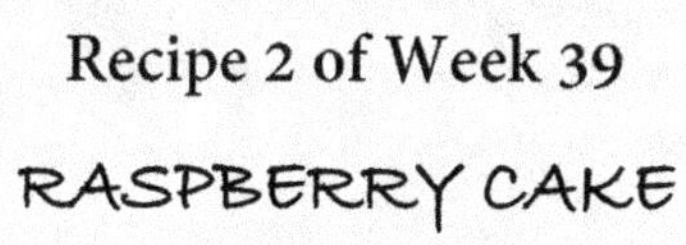

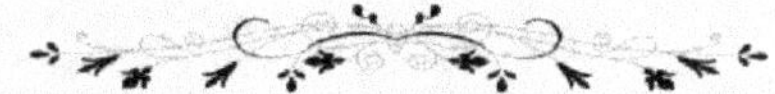

Here is a recipe that combines sweets and fruit and can thus inspire you to create your own variations.

You can also have this healthy cake to honor the feminine energies of your wholeness, regardless of your gender.

Type of Meal	Healthy Snack Dessert
Type of Dish	Lacto-Ovo-Vegetarian Non-Vegetarian
Preparation Time	Approximately 10 minutes Approximately 30 minutes, refrigeration time
Cooking Time	Approximately 35 minutes
Servings	16 pieces
The AilamA® Cookbook advises You	If you want to preserve the flavour of the raspberries, take the cake out of the oven earlier so that the fruit will remain quite firm.

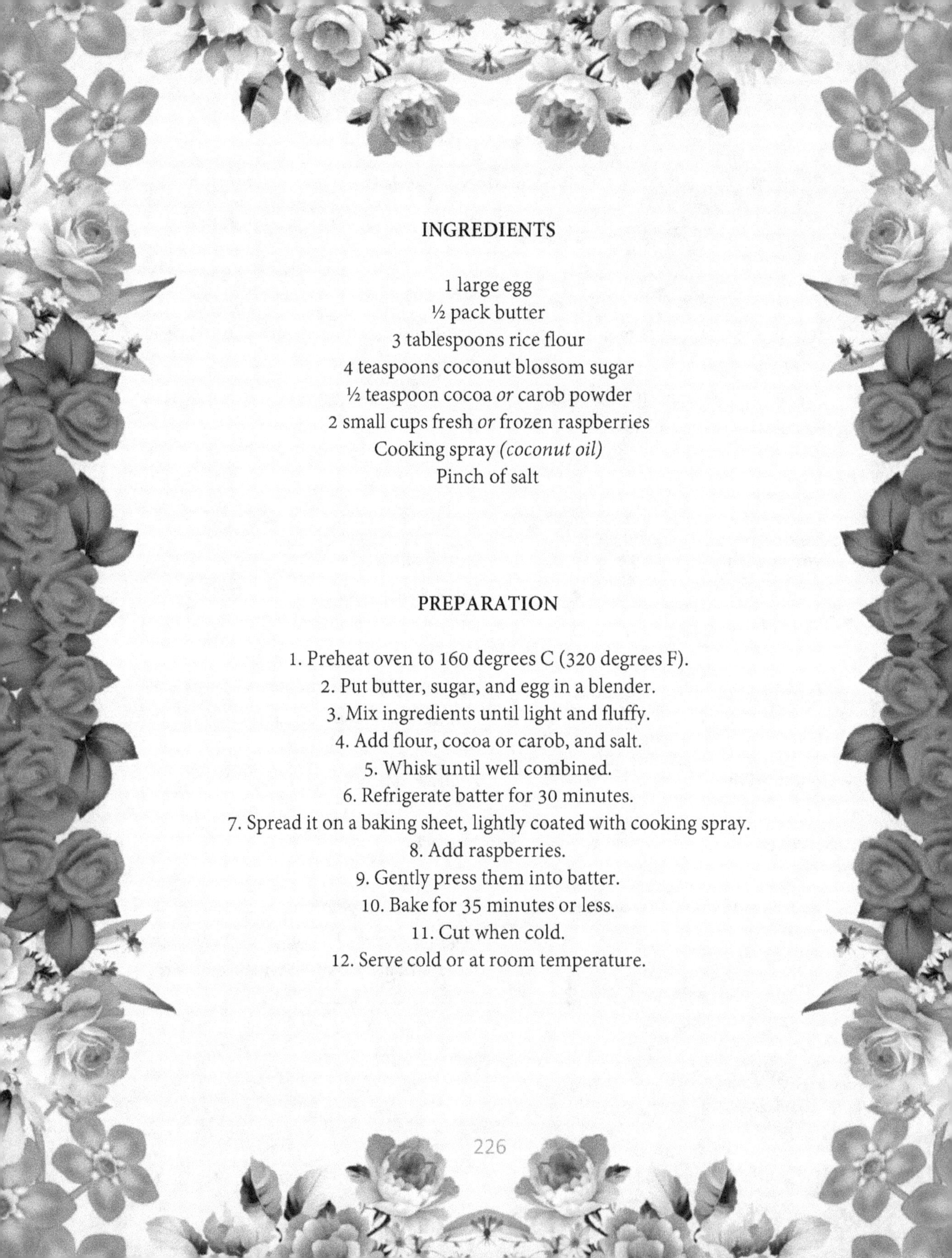

INGREDIENTS

1 large egg
½ pack butter
3 tablespoons rice flour
4 teaspoons coconut blossom sugar
½ teaspoon cocoa *or* carob powder
2 small cups fresh *or* frozen raspberries
Cooking spray *(coconut oil)*
Pinch of salt

PREPARATION

1. Preheat oven to 160 degrees C (320 degrees F).
2. Put butter, sugar, and egg in a blender.
3. Mix ingredients until light and fluffy.
4. Add flour, cocoa or carob, and salt.
5. Whisk until well combined.
6. Refrigerate batter for 30 minutes.
7. Spread it on a baking sheet, lightly coated with cooking spray.
8. Add raspberries.
9. Gently press them into batter.
10. Bake for 35 minutes or less.
11. Cut when cold.
12. Serve cold or at room temperature.

You Matter!

1. Take four gorgeous pictures of your culinary result.

2. Write down your impressions of the recipe.

a. Did you like it?

____

b. Was it difficult?

____

c. Did you find all the ingredients?

____

d. Did you make any changes to the recipe to better suit your dietary needs?

____

____

e. Will you cook it again?

____

f. Will you share it with your family and friends?

____

g. How did it make your body feel?

____

____

h. How were you feeling before cooking the recipe?

____

____

i. How were you feeling after eating the culinary result?

____

____

The Recipe of Week 40
MIXED SALAD

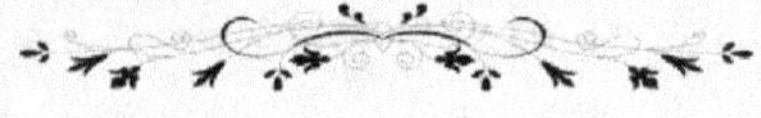

Here is yet another healthy salad for you and your family.

You can also have it when you feel guilty about something you have done to someone.

Type of Meal	Snack
	Main Course
Type of Dish	Vegetarian
	Non-Vegetarian
Preparation Time	Approximately 5 minutes
	Approximately 20 minutes, boiling time
	Approximately 20 minutes, broiling time
	Approximately 30 minutes, soaking time
Cooking Time	Approximately 30 minutes
Servings	4
The AilamA® Cookbook advises You	You can either bake or broil zucchini to get a similar taste and texture. You can place them sliced or halved on the grill or in the oven.

INGREDIENTS

2 moderate red beets, moderately diced
2 moderate zucchini, halved lengthwise, thinly sliced
3 moderate sweet red peppers
1 handful seaweed, previously soaked in spring water
4 tablespoons fresh parsley, including stems, washed and chopped
4 tablespoons extra virgin olive oil
¼ cup (germinated) walnuts, coarsely ground
¼ cup (germinated) almonds, coarsely ground
½ moderate lemon, juiced *(optional)*
½ teaspoon unrefined rock salt

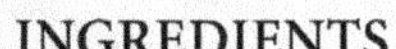

PREPARATION

1. Boil beets and beans separately for at least 20 minutes.
2. Broil zucchini and sweet red peppers until soft yet not mushy.
3. Peel red peppers.
4. Cut red peppers into moderate-sized pieces.
5. Transfer to a mixing bowl.
3. Add parsley, oil, salt, almonds, and walnuts.
4. Mix well.
5. Add lemon juice for a sweet-sour taste. *(optional)*
6. Serve with meats or by itself.

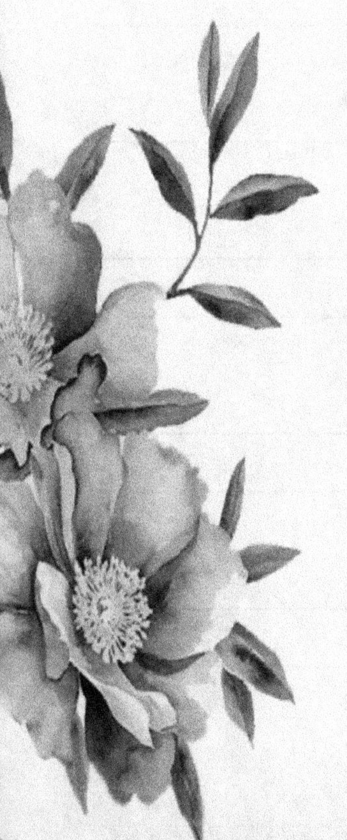

You Matter!

1. Take four gorgeous pictures of your culinary result.

2. Write down your impressions of the recipe.

a. Did you like it?

____

b. Was it difficult?

____

c. Did you find all the ingredients?

____

d. Did you make any changes to the recipe to better suit your dietary needs?

____

____

e. Will you cook it again?

____

f. Will you share it with your family and friends?

____

g. How did it make your body feel?

____

____

h. How were you feeling before cooking the recipe?

____

____

i. How were you feeling after eating the culinary result?

____

____

PIZZA CHAMELEON

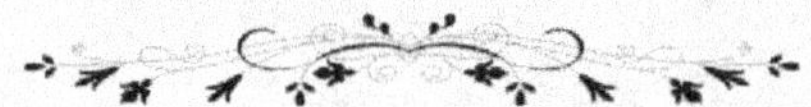

Make your own pizza at home with whatever ingredients you consider beneficial to you. Here is a recipe with very nutritious combinations for both vegetarians and non-vegetarians.

You can also eat this pizza when a certain event has filled you with nostalgia.

Type of Meal	Snack Breakfast Main Course
Type of Dish	Lacto-Ovo-Vegetarian Non-Vegetarian
Preparation Time	Approximately 30 minutes *or* Approximately 1½ hours
Cooking Time	Approximately 30 minutes
Servings	4
The AilamA® Cookbook advises You	If you don't want to toil at kneading or you are too restless to wait for the dough to rise, you can replace the pizza base with slices of healthy (homemade) bread. Make sure they fit the pizza pan perfectly so that the topping will stay in place while baking in the oven. *(See also page 63.)*

INGREDIENTS

1 large whole egg
5 egg whites
½ tablespoon coconut blossom sugar
1 teaspoon unrefined sea salt
4 tablespoons rice oil
300 g whole rice flour
100g whole rye flour
1 glass spring water
1 teaspoon dried thyme
3 teaspoons dried oregano
1 teaspoon dried basil
¾ pack fresh yeast *(optional)*
1 medium zucchini, cut small
1 large red pepper, cut small
1 cup kalamata *or* green olives, stone removed, halved
½ cup parmesan *or* diced homemade pressed cheese *(See also page 35.)*
½ cup diced homemade mozzarella *(See also page 283.)*
1 large red onion, moderately diced
2 celery stalks, cut small
1 cup oyster mushrooms, moderately cut
1 cup fresh *or* frozen peas, washed
1 handful fresh *or* frozen broccoli florets, cut moderately
1 can tuna fish in water, cut small *(optional)*
1 cup meat of your choice, previously cooked, diced small *(optional)*
Cooking spray *(rice oil)*

PREPARATION

Pizza dough (1)

1. Put water, sweetener, salt, 1 teaspoon dried oregano, basil, and thyme, 1 egg, 1 egg white, and oil into bread machine's baking pan.
2. Add flour and yeast.
3. Select **Dough** setting.
4. Take dough out of bread machine, when done.
5. Let it rise for 1 hour.
6. Preheat oven to 160 degrees C (320 degrees F).

Crust pizza dough (2)

1. Preheat oven to 160 degrees C (320 degrees F).
2. Put water, sweetener, salt, 1 teaspoon dried oregano, basil, and thyme, 1 egg, 1 egg white, oil, and flour in a large bowl.
3. Knead well with hands.
4. Turn onto a well-floured surface.
5. Knead for 10 minutes.
6. Add more flour when sticky.
7. Coat a pizza pan with cooking spray.
8. Flatten dough into it.
9. Let it rest for a while, covered with a towel.

Pizza topping

1. Mix 3 egg whites with parmesan or pressed cheese or mozzarella.
2. Beat until quite fluffy.
3. Pour content over dough.
4. Spread well.
5. Top with zucchini, pepper, celery stalk, olives, mushrooms, broccoli, and peas.
6. Sprinkle with oregano.
7. Cook for 30 minutes or so.
8. Keep an eye on it.
9. Add fish or meat 5 minutes before taking it out. *(non-vegetarian dish)*
10. Serve it hot or warm.

You Matter!

1. Take four gorgeous pictures of your culinary result.

2. Write down your impressions of the recipe.

a. Did you like it?

____

b. Was it difficult?

____

c. Did you find all the ingredients?

____

d. Did you make any changes to the recipe to better suit your dietary needs?

____

____

e. Will you cook it again?

____

f. Will you share it with your family and friends?

____

g. How did it make your body feel?

____

____

h. How were you feeling before cooking the recipe?

____

____

i. How were you feeling after eating the culinary result?

____

____

CHICO-TEA

Here is an invigorating beverage that combines the strengths of two healthy plants for a much-needed energy boost.

You can drink it at the beginning of a new project to seal your enthusiasm for the upcoming work.

Type of Meal	Snack
Type of Dish	Vegetarian Non-Vegetarian
Preparation Time	Approximately 2 minutes
Cooking Time	Approximately 5 minutes
Servings	1 cup
The AilamA® Cookbook advises You	This healthy coffee will have a sour touch to its bitter-sweet taste because of the large amount of vitamin C in rose hips.

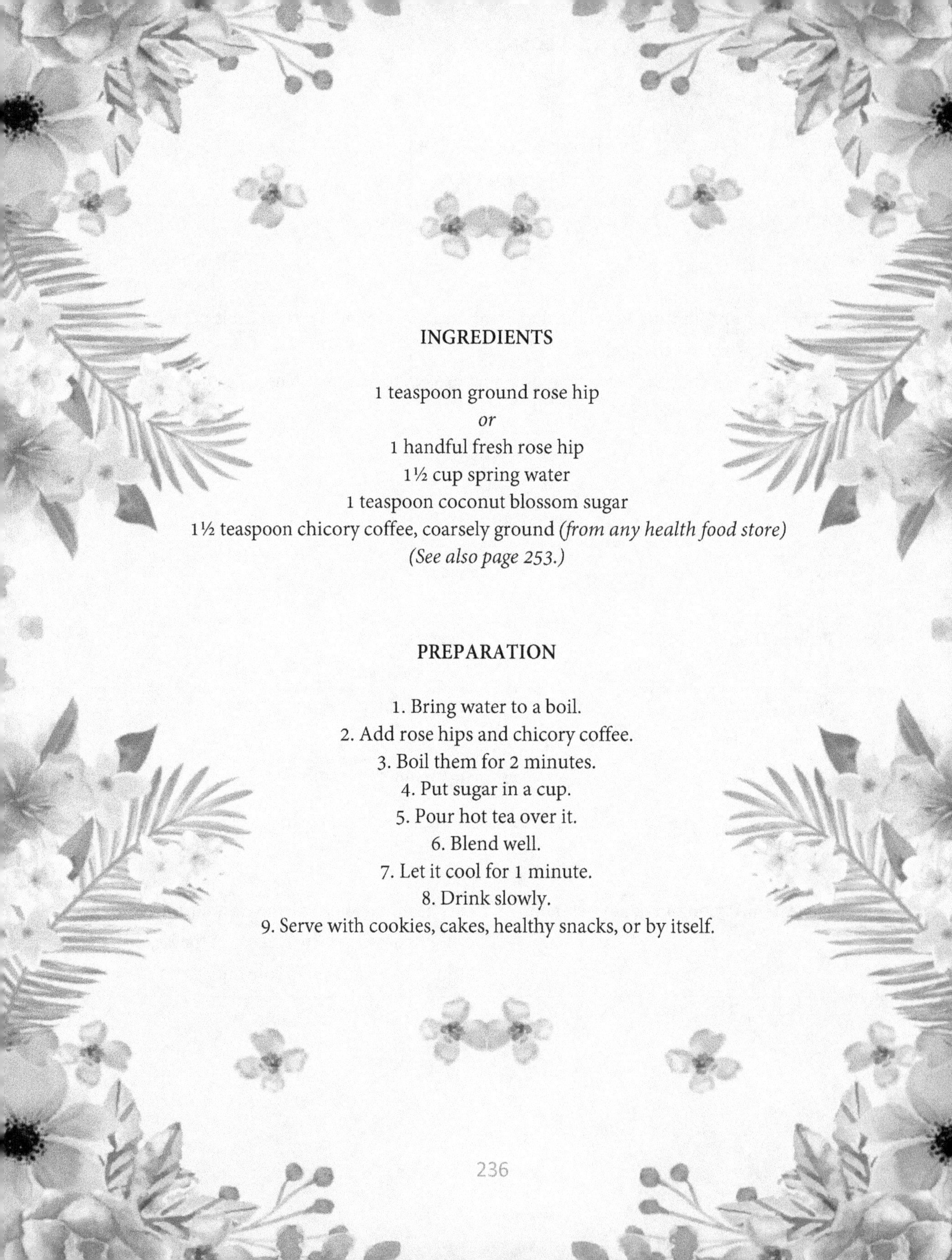

INGREDIENTS

1 teaspoon ground rose hip
or
1 handful fresh rose hip
1½ cup spring water
1 teaspoon coconut blossom sugar
1½ teaspoon chicory coffee, coarsely ground *(from any health food store)*
(See also page 253.)

PREPARATION

1. Bring water to a boil.
2. Add rose hips and chicory coffee.
3. Boil them for 2 minutes.
4. Put sugar in a cup.
5. Pour hot tea over it.
6. Blend well.
7. Let it cool for 1 minute.
8. Drink slowly.
9. Serve with cookies, cakes, healthy snacks, or by itself.

You Matter!

1. Take four gorgeous pictures of your culinary result.

2. Write down your impressions of the recipe.

a. Did you like it?

____

b. Was it difficult?

____

c. Did you find all the ingredients?

____

d. Did you make any changes to the recipe to better suit your dietary needs?

____

____

e. Will you cook it again?

____

f. Will you share it with your family and friends?

____

g. How did it make your body feel?

____

____

h. How were you feeling before cooking the recipe?

____

____

i. How were you feeling after eating the culinary result?

____

____

MACROBIOTIC SOUP

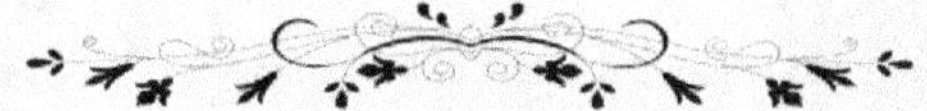

Soups and broths are a great delight in all seasons. Here is another healthy recipe for you and your family.

You can also enjoy this soup whenever you look back on your career with great satisfaction.

Type of Meal	Main Course
	Appetizer
Type of Dish	Pesco-Ovo-Vegetarian
	Non-Vegetarian
Preparation Time	Approximately 5 minutes
Cooking Time	Approximately 45 minutes
Servings	4
The AilamA® Cookbook advises You	Soups can also be eaten alone, packed with nutrients as they are.

INGREDIENTS

2 egg whites
1 zucchini, moderately cut
1½ cups green peas, washed
1 handful string beans, washed, halved
1 handful seaweed, previously soaked in water
1 handful oyster mushrooms, washed, moderately cut
2 teaspoons unrefined rock salt
2 teaspoons mixed herbs of your choice *(See also page 6.)*
1 can tuna fish in water *(non-vegetarian dish)*

PREPARATION

1. Put water and vegetables into a pot.
2. Bring to a boil.
3. Cover with lid.
4. Boil over low heat for 30 minutes.
5. Add salt, herbs, and egg whites.
6. Stir gently.
7. Let it cool for 2 minutes.
8. Add fish. *(non-vegetarian dish)*
9. Stir one last time.
10. Serve hot, warm, or at room temperature.

You Matter!

1. Take four gorgeous pictures of your culinary result.

2. Write down your impressions of the recipe.

a. Did you like it?

____

b. Was it difficult?

____

c. Did you find all the ingredients?

____

d. Did you make any changes to the recipe to better suit your dietary needs?

____

____

e. Will you cook it again?

____

f. Will you share it with your family and friends?

____

g. How did it make your body feel?

____

____

h. How were you feeling before cooking the recipe?

____

____

i. How were you feeling after eating the culinary result?

____

____

MINCED MIX

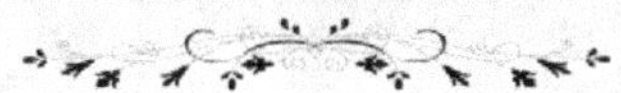

This mixture can be used for meatballs, fish balls, burgers, meat tarts, and even homemade sausages.

If you are a vegetarian, it is also perfect for your veggie burgers or veggie balls and pies.

You can also binge on these goodies after having gotten the promotion you have wanted for such a long time.

Type of Meal	Main Course Snack Dinner
Type of Dish	Vegetarian Pesco-Vegetarian Non-Vegetarian
Preparation Time	Approximately 45 minutes
Cooking Time	Approximately 30 minutes
Servings	8
The AilamA® Cookbook advises You	You can improvise with this mix by adding or subtracting its ingredients as desired.

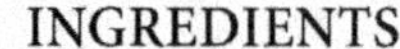

INGREDIENTS

1 large zucchini, moderately cut
2 large red peppers, moderately cut
1 handful string beans, washed, halved
2 celery stalks, moderately cut
2 red onions, moderately cut
8 cloves garlic, peeled
1 bunch fresh parsley, washed
1 bunch fresh dill, washed
½ celery root, moderately cut
1 large carrot, moderately cut
2 large parsnips, moderately cut
3 eggs
2 teaspoons unrefined sea salt
3 teaspoons mixed herbs of your choice *(See also page 6.)*
Meat *or* Fish of your choice *(non-vegetarian dish)*

PREPARATION

1. Mince all vegetable ingredients.
2. Mince meat or fish. *(non-vegetarian dish)*
3. Transfer mixture to a large bowl.
4. Add salt and seasonings.
5. Mix very well.
6. Let it settle for 2 minutes.
7. Use mixture for broiling or baking in oven.

You Matter!

1. Take four gorgeous pictures of your culinary result.

2. Write down your impressions of the recipe.

a. Did you like it?

____

b. Was it difficult?

____

c. Did you find all the ingredients?

____

d. Did you make any changes to the recipe to better suit your dietary needs?

____

____

e. Will you cook it again?

____

f. Will you share it with your family and friends?

____

g. How did it make your body feel?

____

____

h. How were you feeling before cooking the recipe?

____

____

i. How were you feeling after eating the culinary result?

____

____

BAKED APPLES

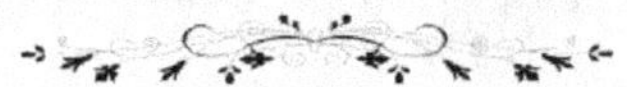

Organic apples are one of the healthiest fruits on the planet. If you've never baked them before, you'll be in for a great culinary surprise.

You can also eat them thus prepared all year around, but especially when you miss a very dear old friend or when you feel lonely.

Type of Meal	Snack
	Dessert
Type of Dish	Vegetarian
	Non-Vegetarian
Preparation Time	Approximately 1 minute
Cooking Time	Approximately 40 minutes
Servings	6
The AilamA® Cookbook advises You	The varieties of apples best suited for baking are said to be Rome Beauty, Jonagold, and Golden Delicious, but you can use any type you want, including Ginger Gold, Golden Delicious, and even Granny Smith. The delicious sweet juice that remains in the pan after baking the apples can sweeten the milk thistle, the chicory-root, or the dandelion-root coffee. *(See also pages 85 and 253.)*

INGREDIENTS

6 organic apples, washed
½ teaspoon ground cinnamon *(optional)*
2 teaspoons seeds of your choice, crushed or whole *(optional)*
2 teaspoons nuts of your choice, crushed *(optional)*
2 teaspoons carob cream *(optional)*
(See also page 50.)

PREPARATION

1. Preheat oven to 190 degrees C (375 degrees F).
2. Put apples in glass baking dish.
3. Bake apples for 40 minutes or so, until soft and golden brown.
4. Bake apples longer if a mushy, pie-filling consistency is desired.
5. Remove apples from oven.
6. Put apples on a platter.
7. Cut in halves, if possible.
8. If mushy, find places where pulp and skin are separated.
9. Sprinkle ground cinnamon over. *(optional)*
10. Serve hot, warm, or at room temperature.
11. Serve with nuts, seeds, or carob cream. *(optional)*

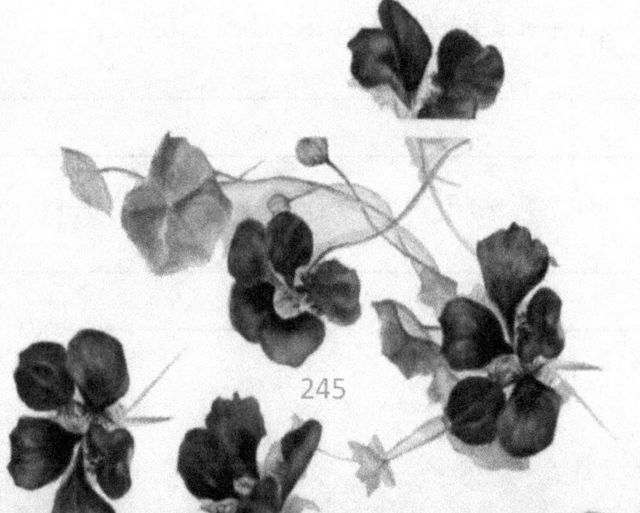

You Matter!

1. Take four gorgeous pictures of your culinary result.

2. Write down your impressions of the recipe.

a. Did you like it?

____

b. Was it difficult?

____

c. Did you find all the ingredients?

____

d. Did you make any changes to the recipe to better suit your dietary needs?

____

____

e. Will you cook it again?

____

f. Will you share it with your family and friends?

____

g. How did it make your body feel?

____

____

h. How were you feeling before cooking the recipe?

____

____

i. How were you feeling after eating the culinary result?

____

____

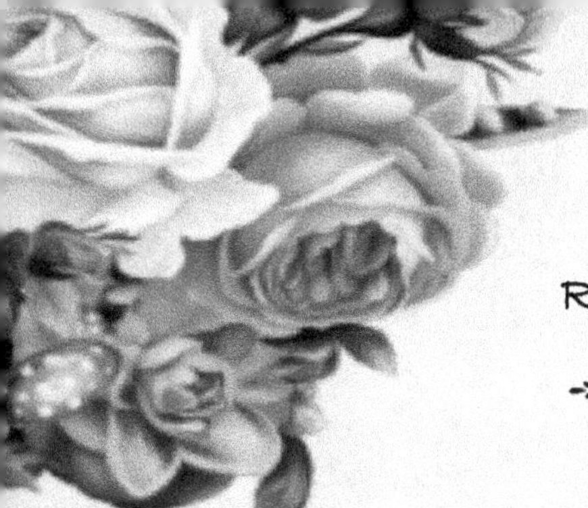

RED PEPPER DIPPING SAUCE

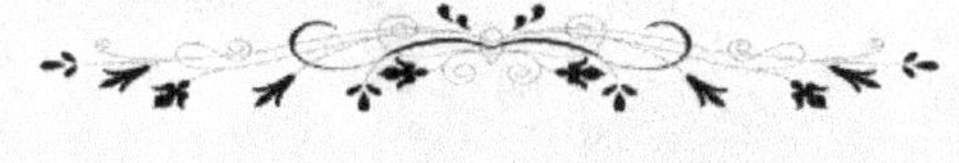

Here is a dish that can be used as a dip, a dressing, or a marinade. If made a little bit thicker, it can be spread on homemade bread or toast.

You can also eat it late at night when working hard on a certain project or when self-disliking thoughts don't let you sleep.

Type of Meal	Snack
	Main Course
Type of Dish	Vegetarian
	Non-Vegetarian
Preparation Time	Approximately 5 minutes
	Approximately 10 minutes, baking time
Cooking Time	Approximately 10 minutes
Servings	3 cups
The AilamA® Cookbook advises You	The consistency of this dish depends on the type of food you want to combine it with. If a dressing, add more water. It's entirely up to you.

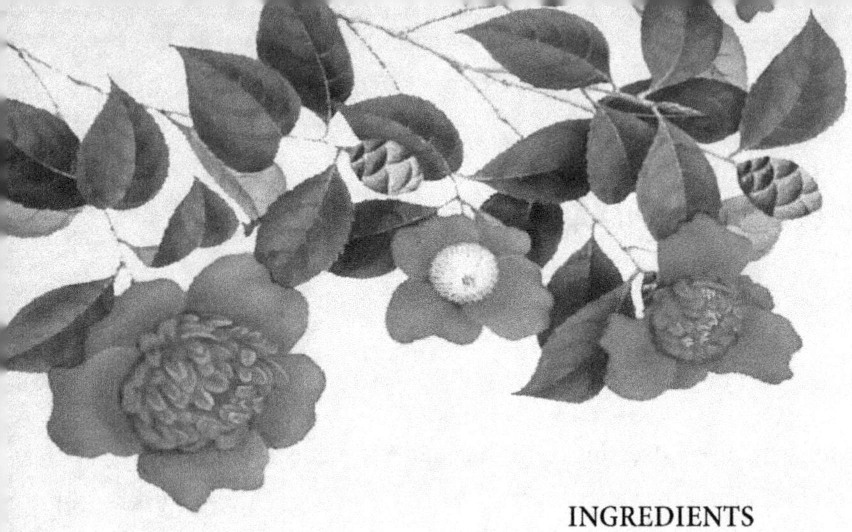

INGREDIENTS

1 egg
1 large red pepper, coarsely cut
1 medium onion, previously baked
1 cup extra virgin olive oil
1 moderate lemon, juiced
1 cup spring water *(optional)*
1 tablespoon fresh parsley, washed and chopped
½ teaspoon mixed herbs of your choice *(See also page 6.)*

PREPARATION

1. Blend pepper, oil, and lemon until smooth.
2. Add onion, salt, spices.
3. Blend until smooth.
4. Add water until desired consistency is achieved. *(optional)*
5. Transfer to a mixing bowl.
6. Add parsley.
7. Whisk it until smooth, as desired.
8. Serve with vegetables, salads, or meats.

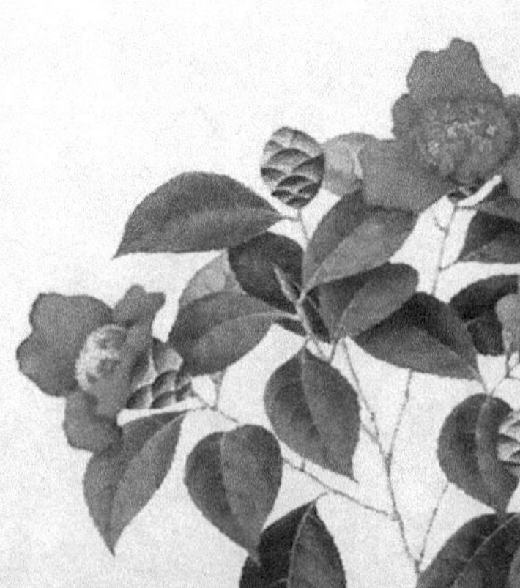

You Matter!

1. Take four gorgeous pictures of your culinary result.

2. Write down your impressions of the recipe.

a. Did you like it?

____

b. Was it difficult?

____

c. Did you find all the ingredients?

____

d. Did you make any changes to the recipe to better suit your dietary needs?

____

____

e. Will you cook it again?

____

f. Will you share it with your family and friends?

____

g. How did it make your body feel?

____

____

h. How were you feeling before cooking the recipe?

____

____

i. How were you feeling after eating the culinary result?

____

____

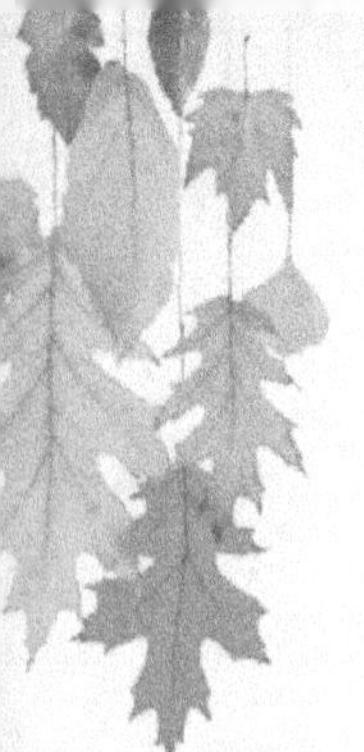

PRUNE CAKE

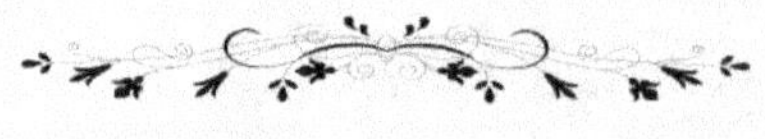

Here is a sugar-free cake for you and your family.

You can also enjoy it along with your friends on a sunny picnic day.

Type of Meal	Snack Dessert
Type of Dish	Ovo-Vegetarian Non-Vegetarian
Preparation Time	Approximately 10 minutes
Cooking Time	Approximately 1 hour
Servings	16 pieces
The AilamA® Cookbook advises You	If cream is too hard, you can add some spring water, or even some of your favourite tea. It has to be creamy yet quite runny at the same time. If you decide to use dates, keep in mind that they are much sweeter than prunes.

INGREDIENTS

10 egg whites
1 handful dried prunes *or* dates
½ cup (germinated) walnuts *or* almonds
Cooking spray *(coconut oil)*
Pinch of salt

PREPARATION

1. Preheat oven to 160 degrees C (320 degrees F).
2. Put dates or prunes and egg whites in a blender.
3. Mix until creamy.
4. Add walnuts or almonds and salt.
5. Whisk until well combined.
6. Pour creamy content into a baking pot, lightly coated with cooking spray.
7. Put baking pot in a larger pot with water.
8. Bake for about 1 hour.
9. Remove from oven.
10. Let it cool.
11. Cut when cold.
12. Serve cold or at room temperature.

You Matter!

1. Take four gorgeous pictures of your culinary result.

2. Write down your impressions of the recipe.

a. Did you like it?

____

b. Was it difficult?

____

c. Did you find all the ingredients?

____

d. Did you make any changes to the recipe to better suit your dietary needs?

____

____

e. Will you cook it again?

____

f. Will you share it with your family and friends?

____

g. How did it make your body feel?

____

____

h. How were you feeling before cooking the recipe?

____

____

i. How were you feeling after eating the culinary result?

____

____

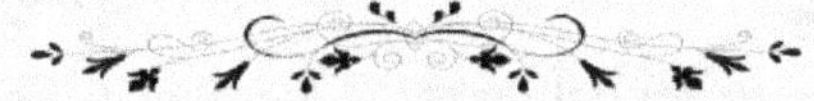

Dandelion roots, like chicory roots, are known as a very potent gallbladder and liver supporter and detoxifier. The best way to introduce them into your everyday diet is by roasting them and then grinding them into a delicious caffeine-free, liver-friendly coffee powder.

Here is the recipe of a beverage that can become your everyday pleasure. You can also drink it whenever you feel tired.

Type of Meal	Snack
Type of Dish	Vegetarian Non-Vegetarian
Preparation Time	Approximately 1 hour, harvesting time Approximately 10 minutes, washing time Approximately 10 minutes, chopping time
Cooking Time	Approximately 15 minutes, roasting time for dried dandelion root Approximately 40 minutes, roasting time for fresh dandelion root
Servings	3 cups
The AilamA® Cookbook advises You	The best season to harvest dandelion roots is early spring. It takes about 15 dandelion roots to make at least 10 small cups of coffee. Make sure you keep them in the oven at the right temperature to come out perfect: dry and toasted, not burned. You can also make chicory coffee from roasted chicory roots following the same recipe.

INGREDIENTS

30 dandelion roots, freshly harvested
or
1 pack dried dandelion roots, organic *(from any health food store)*

PREPARATION

1. Harvest dandelion roots.
or
Buy dried dandelion roots.
2. Wash roots thoroughly.
3. Separate the smaller, thinner parts. *(optional)*
4. Roast fresh or dried dandelion roots at moderate temperature. (177 degrees C *or* 350 degrees F)
5. Stir roots occasionally, until they become completely dry and brown (not scorched).
6. Let roots cool.
7. Eat roots whole, 1 teaspoonful 2 times a day.
8. Grind roots into coarse powder.

Coffee

1. Bring 1¼ cups spring water to a boil.
2. Add ½ teaspoon milk thistle coffee.
3. Simmer for 5 minutes.
4. Strain it through a fine mesh strainer.
5. Drink it hot, warm, or cold.
6. Drink it black.
7. Drink it with coconut water and/or coconut milk. *(optional)*
8. Drink it with the juice from baked apples. *(optional)*
(See also page 244.)

You Matter!

1. Take four gorgeous pictures of your culinary result.

2. Write down your impressions of the recipe.

a. Did you like it?

____

b. Was it difficult?

____

c. Did you find all the ingredients?

____

d. Did you make any changes to the recipe to better suit your dietary needs?

____

____

e. Will you cook it again?

____

f. Will you share it with your family and friends?

____

g. How did it make your body feel?

____

____

h. How were you feeling before cooking the recipe?

____

____

i. How were you feeling after eating the culinary result?

____

____

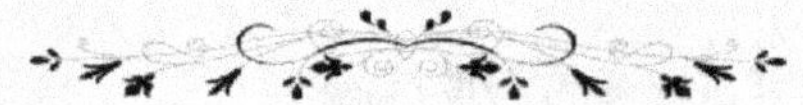

Here is yet another easy sushi recipe for you and your family.
You can also serve this dish when you host a dinner party where there will be
people who dislike eating raw fish.

Type of Meal	Main Course
	Appetizer
	Snack
Type of Dish	Pesco-Vegetarian
	Non-Vegetarian
Preparation Time	Approximately 10 minutes
	Approximately 20 minutes, boiling time
Cooking Time	Approximately 20 minutes
Servings	4
The AilamA® Cookbook advises You	Quinoa can successfully replace rice in sushi recipes. Another healthy option is millet.

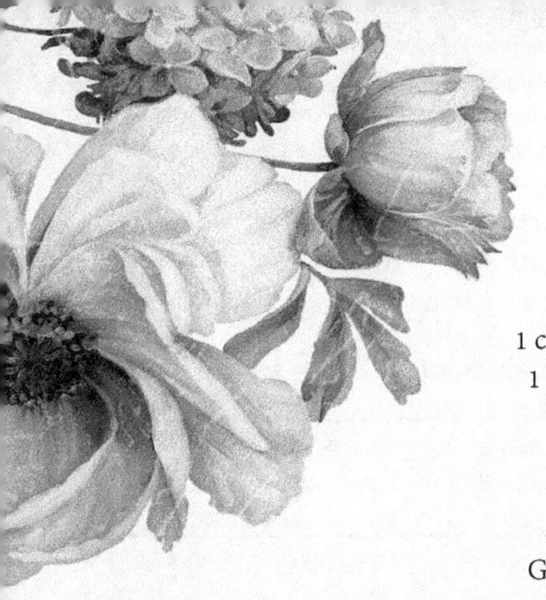

INGREDIENTS

2 sheets nori seaweed
1 cup quinoa *or* millet, previously boiled
1 large strip tuna fish, canned in water
2 long strips red pepper
1 lemon, juiced
1 strip green salad
Pinch of unrefined rock salt
Grated horseradish, pickled *(optional)*
Fresh ginger, grated *(optional)*

PREPARATION

1. Put quinoa or millet in a pot.
2. Cover it with spring water
3. Add pinch of salt.
4. Bring quinoa or millet to a boil.
5. Let it simmer until done.
6. Sprinkle it with sesame oil.
7. Mix well.
8. Let quinoa or millet get cold.
9. Position nori seaweed on a bamboo sushi mat.
10. Spread a thin or thick layer of quinoa or millet, as desired.
11. Add fish, pepper, and salad.
12. Sprinkle with salt and lemon.
13. Roll to form sushi.
14. Slice with a sharp knife.
15. Serve with pickled horseradish or fresh ginger on top.

You Matter!

1. Take four gorgeous pictures of your culinary result.

2. Write down your impressions of the recipe.

a. Did you like it?

____

b. Was it difficult?

____

c. Did you find all the ingredients?

____

d. Did you make any changes to the recipe to better suit your dietary needs?

____

____

e. Will you cook it again?

____

f. Will you share it with your family and friends?

____

g. How did it make your body feel?

____

____

h. How were you feeling before cooking the recipe?

____

____

i. How were you feeling after eating the culinary result?

____

____

The Recipe of Week 47
VEGGIE CREAM

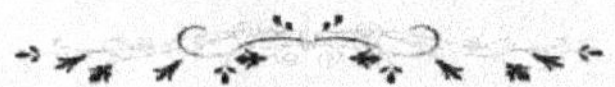

Here is the recipe of a tasty creamed soup for you and your family.
It is also perfect for hot weather, so feel free to eat this soup anytime you want to
chill out during the summer months.

Type of Meal	Main Course Appetizer
Type of Dish	Vegetarian Non-Vegetarian
Preparation Time	Approximately 10 minutes
Cooking Time	Approximately 45 minutes
Servings	4
The AilamA® Cookbook advises You	Oyster mushrooms have the texture and taste of chicken breast, so you can (sometimes) replace one type of protein with the other, even if you are a meat-eater.

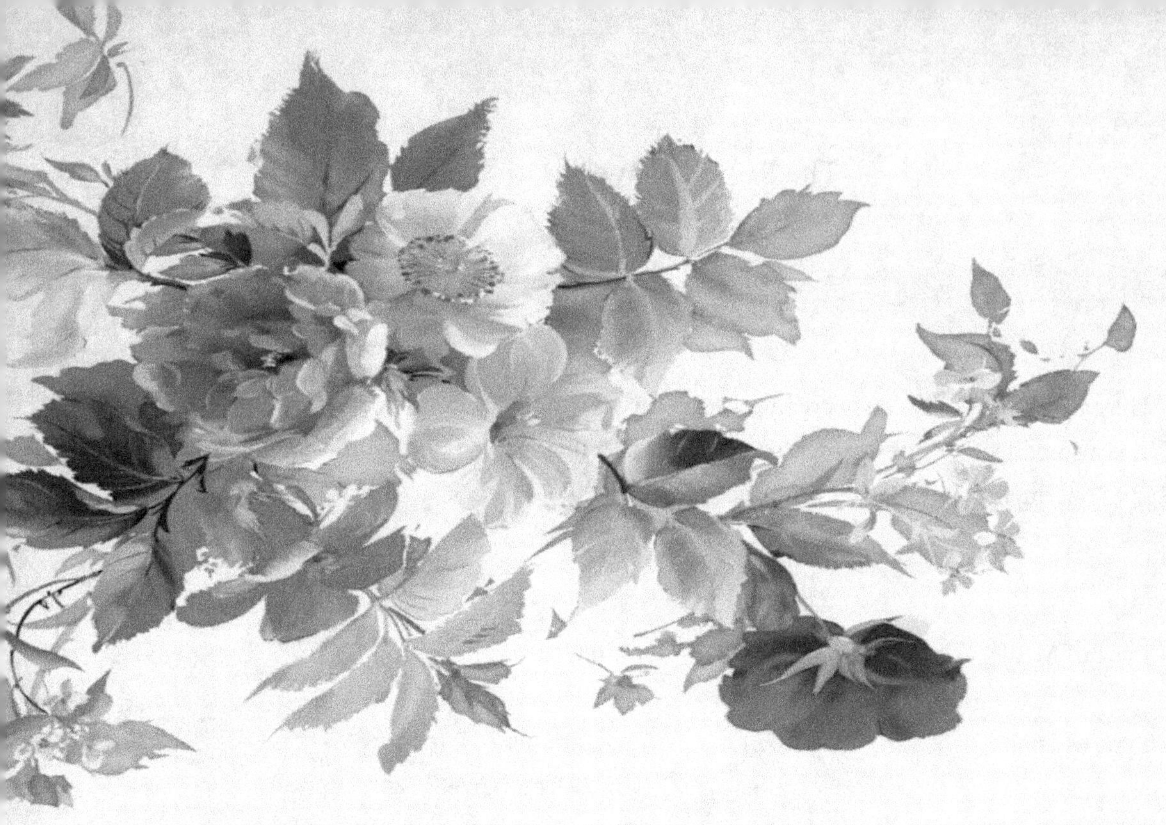

INGREDIENTS

2 handfuls oyster *or* portobello mushrooms, thinly sliced lengthwise
½ handful broccoli florets, washed, halved
½ cup peas, washed
2 large parsnips, largely cut
1 moderate carrot, largely cut
2 onions, halved
1 zucchini, largely cut
1 egg
1 bunch fresh parsley, washed and chopped
Chicken *or* hen *or* cock *or* turkey stock *(non-vegetarian dish)*
Chicken *or* hen *or* cock *or* turkey breast, previously cooked *(non-vegetarian dish)*
2 teaspoons unrefined sea salt
2 teaspoons mixed herbs of your choice *(See also page 6.)*

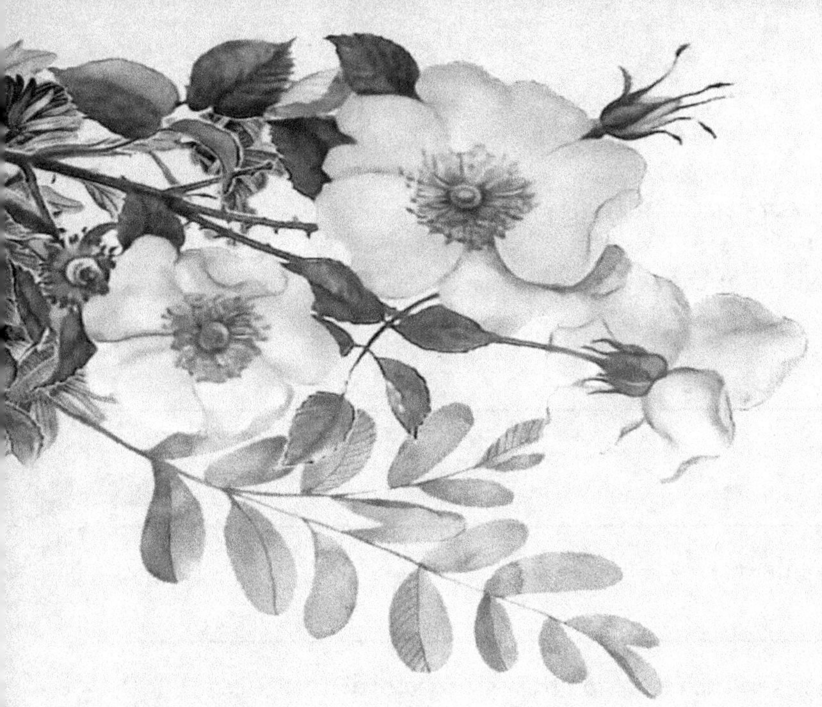

PREPARATION

1. Put stock or water and vegetables into a pot.

2. Bring to a boil.

3. Cover with lid.

4. Boil over low heat.

5. Take mushrooms out after 10 minutes.

6. Let mushrooms cool.

7. Continue to boil the rest for another 20 minutes.

8. Let it cool.

9. Transfer all to a blender bowl.

10. Mix well with 2 cups veggie stock or water or meat stock.

11. Add salt and herbs.

12. Add egg and breast. *(non-vegetarian dish)*

13. Blend well.

14. Let it cool for 2 minutes.

15. Transfer mixture back to pot.

16. Stir again.

17. Serve hot, warm, or at room temperature, with freshly chopped parsley.

You Matter!

1. Take four gorgeous pictures of your culinary result.

2. Write down your impressions of the recipe.

a. Did you like it?

____

b. Was it difficult?

____

c. Did you find all the ingredients?

____

d. Did you make any changes to the recipe to better suit your dietary needs?

____

____

e. Will you cook it again?

____

f. Will you share it with your family and friends?

____

g. How did it make your body feel?

____

____

h. How were you feeling before cooking the recipe?

____

____

i. How were you feeling after eating the culinary result?

____

____

SALMON-CHICKEN SALAD

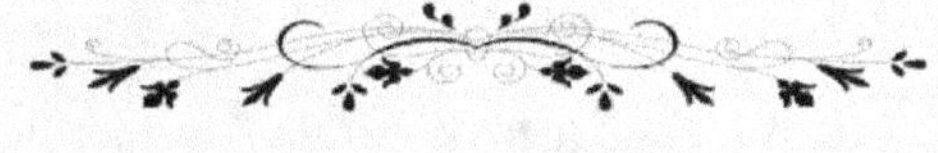

Here is a tasty salad for you and your family, if you are a non-vegetarian.
It can also become your comfort food after a fit of good, liberating crying.

Type of Meal	Main Course
	Snack
Type of Dish	Non-Vegetarian
Preparation Time	Approximately 10 minutes
	Approximately 8 minutes, broiling time
Cooking Time	Approximately 8 minutes
Servings	4
The AilamA® Cookbook advises You	You can slice your chicken breast very thinly before broiling it. In this way, less cooking time will be needed while the breast will remain juicy and tender.

INGREDIENTS

3 turnip cabbages (kohlrabi), moderately grated
3 red beets, moderately grated
1 onion, moderately diced, previously baked
2 tablespoons extra virgin olive oil
1 bunch fresh parsley, washed and chopped
1 raw fresh salmon fillet, cut into moderate pieces
3 chicken breasts, broiled, cut into moderate pieces
½ lemon, juiced
¼ teaspoon unrefined rock salt

PREPARATION

1. Mix all ingredients in a glass bowl.
2. Sprinkle with oil, salt, and lemon.
3. Blend well.
4. Serve at room temperature or chilled.

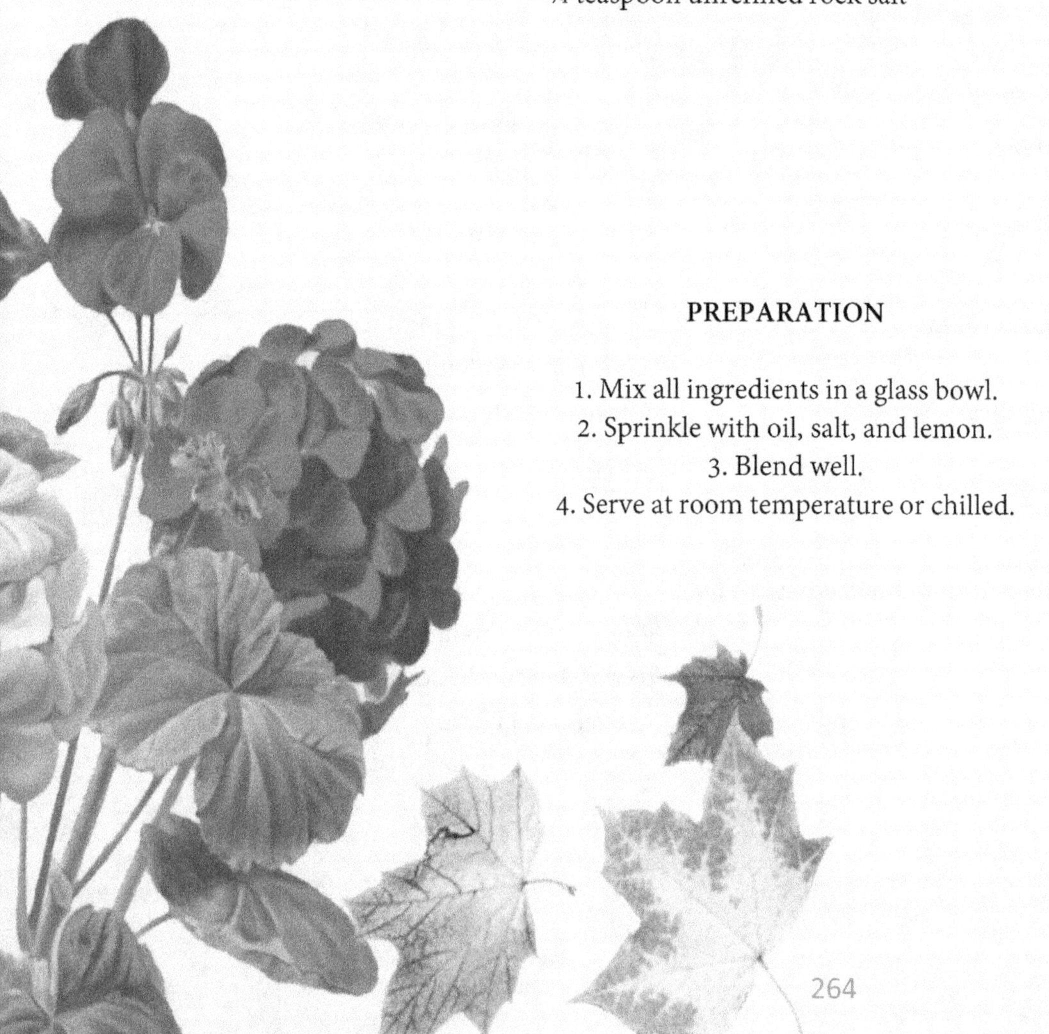

You Matter!

1. Take four gorgeous pictures of your culinary result.

2. Write down your impressions of the recipe.

a. Did you like it?

____

b. Was it difficult?

____

c. Did you find all the ingredients?

____

d. Did you make any changes to the recipe to better suit your dietary needs?

____

____

e. Will you cook it again?

____

f. Will you share it with your family and friends?

____

g. How did it make your body feel?

____

____

h. How were you feeling before cooking the recipe?

____

____

i. How were you feeling after eating the culinary result?

____

____

CHOCOLATE SWEET DELIGHT

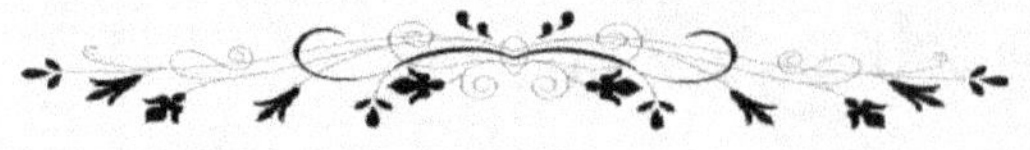

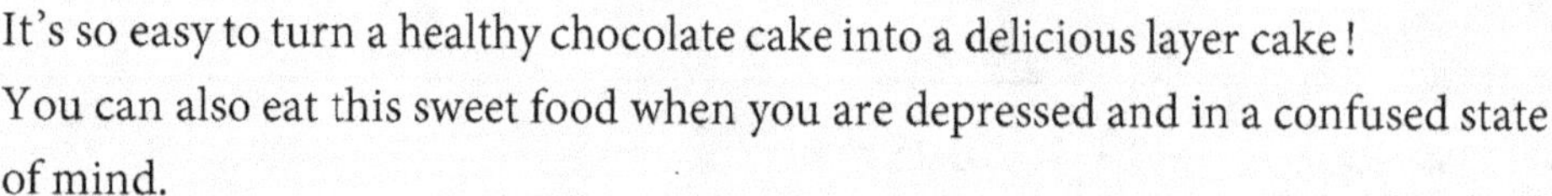

It's so easy to turn a healthy chocolate cake into a delicious layer cake!
You can also eat this sweet food when you are depressed and in a confused state
of mind.

Type of Meal	Snack
	Dessert
Type of Dish	Lacto-Ovo-Vegetarian
	Non-Vegetarian
Preparation Time	Approximately 10 minutes
Cooking Time	Approximately 1 hour
Servings	6 pieces
The AilamA® Cookbook advises You	Because of its nutrient-dense ingredients, make sure you won't eat too much of the cake at once.

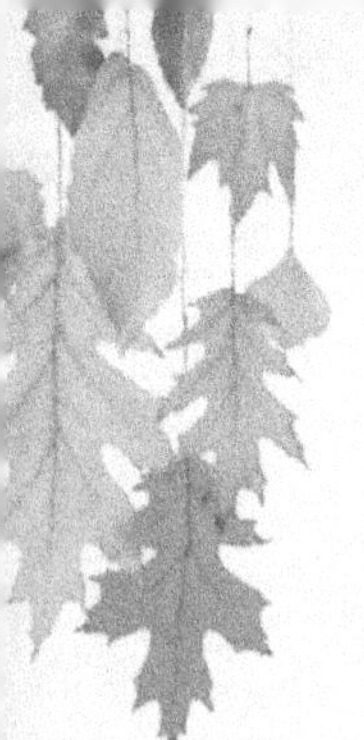

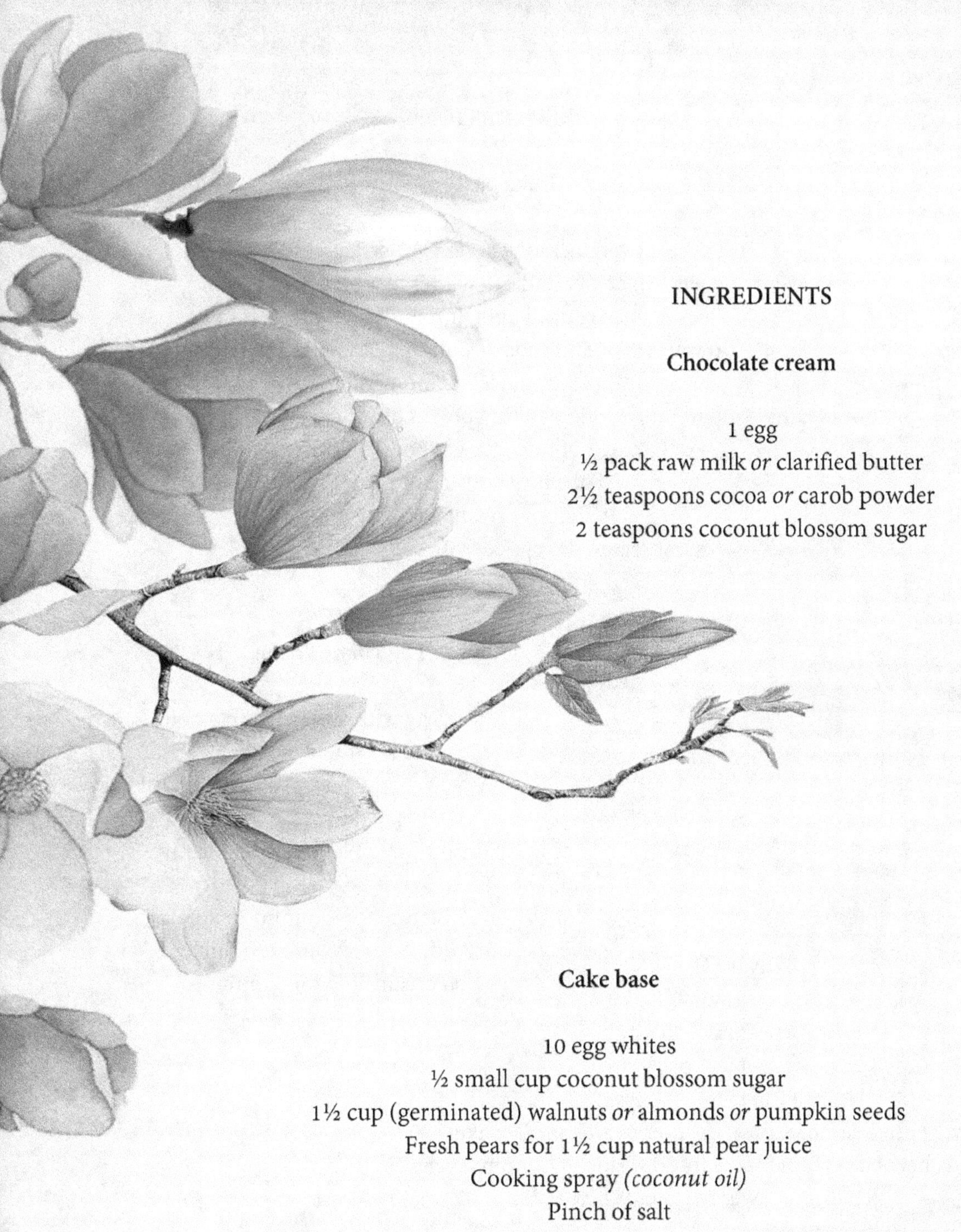

INGREDIENTS

Chocolate cream

1 egg
½ pack raw milk *or* clarified butter
2½ teaspoons cocoa *or* carob powder
2 teaspoons coconut blossom sugar

Cake base

10 egg whites
½ small cup coconut blossom sugar
1½ cup (germinated) walnuts *or* almonds *or* pumpkin seeds
Fresh pears for 1½ cup natural pear juice
Cooking spray *(coconut oil)*
Pinch of salt

PREPARATION

Cake base

1. Preheat oven to 160 degrees C (320 degrees F).
2. Put sweetener and egg whites in a blender.
3. Mix until light and fluffy.
4. Add walnuts or almonds or pumpkin seeds and salt.
5. Whisk until well combined.
6. Pour creamy content into a round baking pot, lightly coated with cooking spray.
7. Put baking pot into a larger pot with water.
8. Bake for about 1 hour.
9. Remove from oven.
10. Prepare pear juice from fresh pears.

Chocolate cream

1. Mix egg with sweetener in a pot.
2. Stir until blended.
3. Set pot in a bain-marie (double boiler).
4. Add butter.
5. Stir until well blended and creamy.
6. Add cocoa or carob powder.
7. Mix well for 1 minute or so.
8. Add spring water if too thick.
9. Let cream cool for 5 minutes.

Layer cake

1. Bring pear juice to a boil.
2. Let it cool.
3. Cut cake into 2 layers.
4. Slowly pour pear juice on each interior side until soaked.
5. Spread chocolate cream on the interior side of bottom layer.
6. Place other layer back to its place.
7. Cover cake in chocolate cream.
8. Cut when cold.
9. Serve chilled or at room temperature.

You Matter!

1. Take four gorgeous pictures of your culinary result.

2. Write down your impressions of the recipe.

a. Did you like it?

____

b. Was it difficult?

____

c. Did you find all the ingredients?

____

d. Did you make any changes to the recipe to better suit your dietary needs?

____

____

e. Will you cook it again?

____

f. Will you share it with your family and friends?

____

g. How did it make your body feel?

____

____

h. How were you feeling before cooking the recipe?

____

____

i. How were you feeling after eating the culinary result?

____

____

COCO COLD

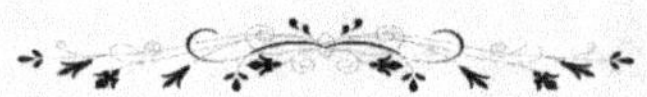

Here is the recipe of one of the simplest and healthiest ice creams ever, for torrid summers and happy holidays.

Also, you can binge on this ice cream when you are bored with something in your life.

Type of Meal	Dessert
	Snack
Type of Dish	Ovo-Vegetarian
	Non-Vegetarian
Preparation Time	Approximately 10 minutes
Cooking Time	Approximately 15 minutes
Servings	6
The AilamA® Cookbook advises You	Instead of figs, macadamia nuts, and sesame seeds, you can create other combinations to suit your own taste. An even simpler variation is just combining coconut water, carob powder, figs, and macadamia nuts, and then place the result (with sesame seeds on top, if so desired) directly in the freezer. This watery version resembles the ice pop or the Popsicle, and it's more liver-friendly.

INGREDIENTS

1 egg
2 tablespoons coconut butter
2 teaspoons carob powder
3 figs (fresh *or* dried), cut into moderate pieces
1 tablespoon (germinated) macadamia nuts, coarsely chopped or blended *(optional)*
1 tablespoon (germinated) sesame seeds, coarsely chopped or blended *(optional)*
1 cup of fresh coconut water, directly from the coconut fruit

PREPARATION

1. Put egg in a pot.
2. Stir egg until well blended.
3. Put pot in a bain-marie (double boiler).
4. Add coconut butter.
5. Stir until well blended and creamy.
6. Add carob powder.
7. Mix well.
8. Add fig pieces.
9. Mix well.
10. Add macadamia nuts. *(optional)*
11. Mix well.
12. Add coconut water.
13. Mix until well blended.
14. Remove pot from heat.
15. Let it cool for 2 minutes.
16. Pour content in small ceramic or glass pots.
17. Sprinkle with sesame seeds. *(optional)*
18. Place in freezer when completely cold.
19. Serve cold or frozen.

You Matter!

1. Take four gorgeous pictures of your culinary result.

2. Write down your impressions of the recipe.

a. Did you like it?

____

b. Was it difficult?

____

c. Did you find all the ingredients?

____

d. Did you make any changes to the recipe to better suit your dietary needs?

____

____

e. Will you cook it again?

____

f. Will you share it with your family and friends?

____

g. How did it make your body feel?

____

____

h. How were you feeling before cooking the recipe?

____

____

i. How were you feeling after eating the culinary result?

____

____

THY STEW

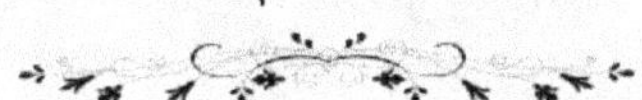

Here is a thyroid-friendly stew recipe, no fat, no tomato juice, just perfect for both vegetarians and non-vegetarians.

You can also have this stew when you feel a deep sadness for all the animals that have to suffer misfortunes.

Type of Meal	Main Course Dinner Supper
Type of Dish	Vegetarian Non-Vegetarian
Preparation Time	Approximately 15 minutes
Cooking Time	Approximately 60 minutes
Servings	12
The AilamA® Cookbook advises You	You can replace mushrooms with string beans to make a differently flavored stew with the same beneficial properties. In both cases, your thyroid will thank you and, along with it, your liver, gallbladder, pancreas, spleen, intestines, and kidneys. If you keep these organs happy, your entire body will stay healthy.

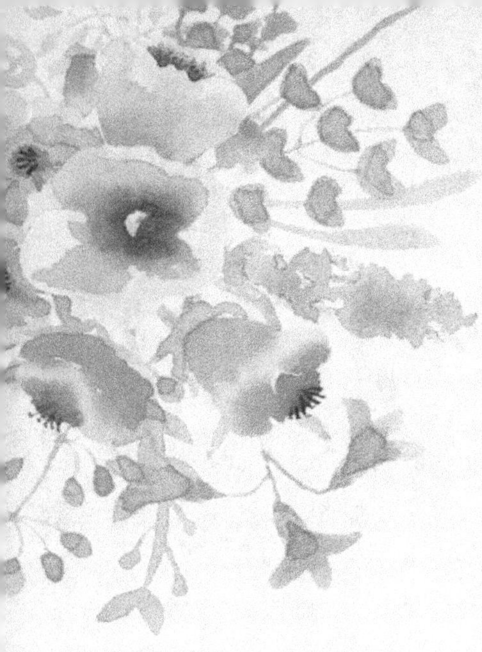

INGREDIENTS

4 large carrots, 2 coarsely grated, 2 halved and cut into moderate pieces
4 medium onions, 2 red, 2 white, roughly chopped
4 handfuls mushrooms of your choice, roughly chopped
3 moderate cups grains of your choice (spelt, oats, barley, rye, rice, etc.),
previously boiled until all scum can be removed
6 chicken thighs (with bones, skinless, all fat removed),
previously boiled until all scum can be removed, roughly cut into moderate pieces,
bones and broth kept for further use *(non-vegetarian dish)*
8 cups spring water *(adjustable quantity)*
8 cups chicken broth *(non-vegetarian dish)*
½ saucerful fresh *or* semi-dried lovage, leaves and stems, roughly chopped
½ saucerful fresh *or* semi-dried parsley, leaves, stems, and roots (if possible), roughly chopped
5 teaspoons dried thyme
1 teaspoon unrefined rock salt

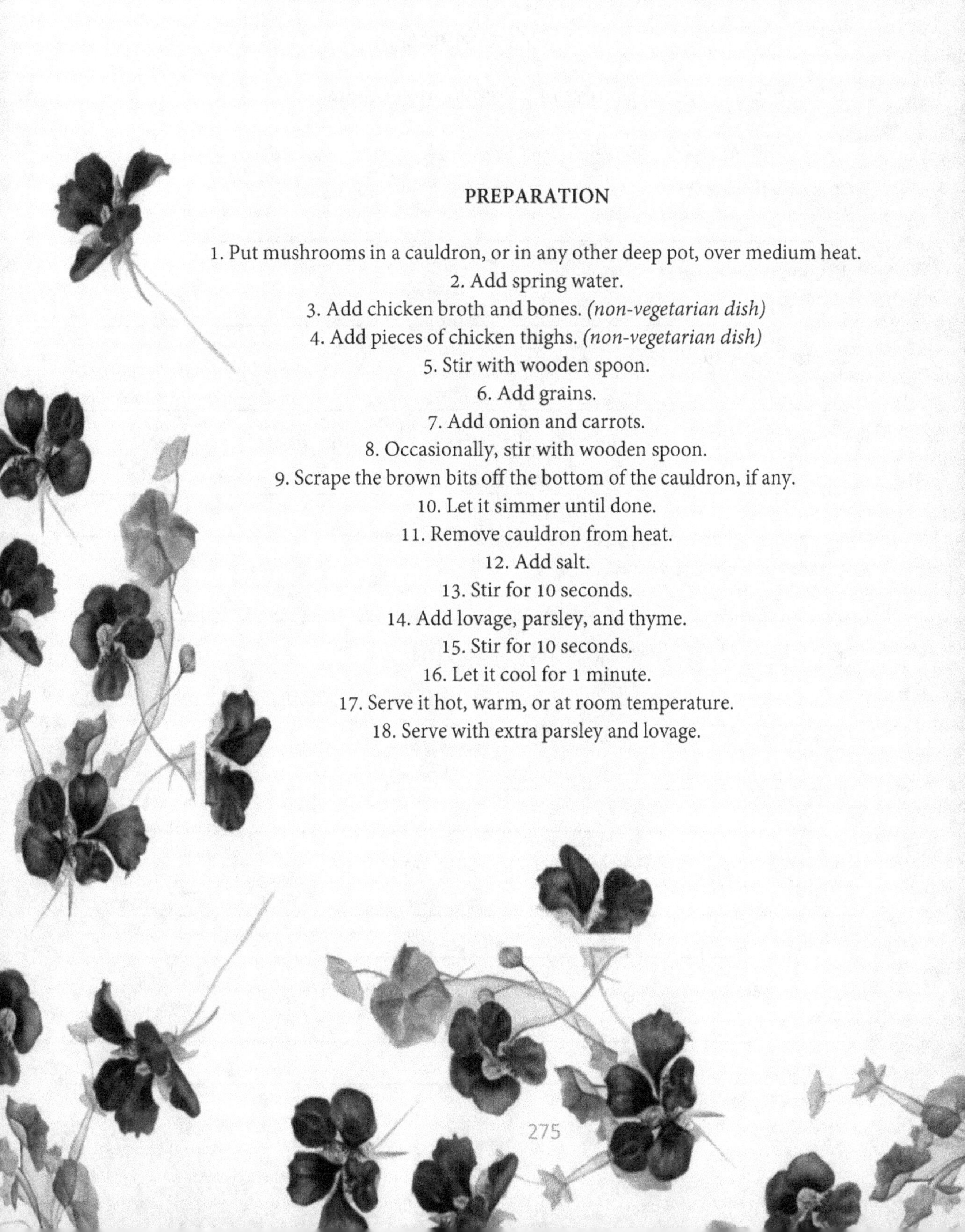

PREPARATION

1. Put mushrooms in a cauldron, or in any other deep pot, over medium heat.
2. Add spring water.
3. Add chicken broth and bones. *(non-vegetarian dish)*
4. Add pieces of chicken thighs. *(non-vegetarian dish)*
5. Stir with wooden spoon.
6. Add grains.
7. Add onion and carrots.
8. Occasionally, stir with wooden spoon.
9. Scrape the brown bits off the bottom of the cauldron, if any.
10. Let it simmer until done.
11. Remove cauldron from heat.
12. Add salt.
13. Stir for 10 seconds.
14. Add lovage, parsley, and thyme.
15. Stir for 10 seconds.
16. Let it cool for 1 minute.
17. Serve it hot, warm, or at room temperature.
18. Serve with extra parsley and lovage.

You Matter!

1. Take four gorgeous pictures of your culinary result.

2. Write down your impressions of the recipe.

a. Did you like it?

____

b. Was it difficult?

____

c. Did you find all the ingredients?

____

d. Did you make any changes to the recipe to better suit your dietary needs?

____

____

e. Will you cook it again?

____

f. Will you share it with your family and friends?

____

g. How did it make your body feel?

____

____

h. How were you feeling before cooking the recipe?

____

____

i. How were you feeling after eating the culinary result?

____

____

MASHED PARSNIPS

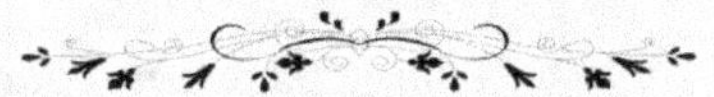

Here is yet another tasty recipe to try. Whether you are a vegetarian or not, this dish is packed with phytonutrients to keep you healthy and fit.

You can also eat it after you have received some unexpected good news.

Type of Meal	Main Course
	Snack
Type of Dish	Ovo-Vegetarian
	Non-Vegetarian
Preparation Time	Approximately 5 minutes
Cooking Time	Approximately 45 minutes
Servings	4
The AilamA® Cookbook advises You	Parsnips taste quite sweet, so they will be twice as rewarding if you are a sweet-toothed person.

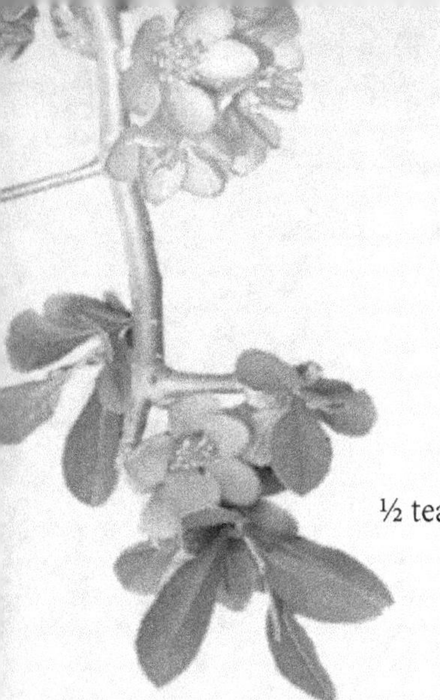

INGREDIENTS

1 egg
8 large parsnips, coarsely cut
1 medium onion, previously baked
1 small cup extra virgin olive oil
½ moderate lemon, juiced *(optional)*
½ teaspoon horseradish, grated, pickled in salt and lemon juice *(See also page 56.)*
1 tablespoon fresh parsley, washed and chopped
¼ teaspoon unrefined rock salt
4 glasses spring water
1½ teaspoons mixed herbs of your choice *(See also page 6.)*

PREPARATION

1. Put parsnips in a pot.
2. Add spring water to cover them.
3. Add 1 teaspoon mixed seasoning.
4. Add horseradish.
5. Boil for 45 minutes or so, until parsnips become soft.
6. Bake onion for 10 minutes.
7. Put boiled parsnips, oil, egg, salt, onion, and mixed herbs in a blender.
8. Blend until smooth or coarsely consistent, as desired.
9. Add lemon juice until desired taste is obtained. *(optional)*
10. Transfer to a mixing bowl.
11. Add parsley.
12. Whisk it until smooth, as desired.
13. Serve hot, warm, or at room temperature.
14. Serve with meats, slices of red pepper, bread, or by itself.

You Matter!

1. Take four gorgeous pictures of your culinary result.

2. Write down your impressions of the recipe.

a. Did you like it?

____

b. Was it difficult?

____

c. Did you find all the ingredients?

____

d. Did you make any changes to the recipe to better suit your dietary needs?

____

____

e. Will you cook it again?

____

f. Will you share it with your family and friends?

____

g. How did it make your body feel?

____

____

h. How were you feeling before cooking the recipe?

____

____

i. How were you feeling after eating the culinary result?

____

____

The Recipe of Week 51
BUCKWHEAT SALAD

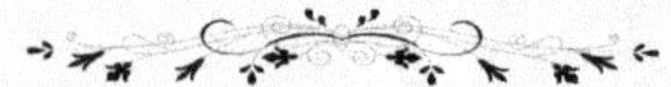

Buckwheat is not really a grain but a gluten-free seed. When soaked in water, buckwheat grains open like small flower buds.

Here is a tasty salad prepared with this wonderful ingredient.

You can also eat it when you study for a difficult exam or when you work hard to achieve a dream.

Type of Meal	Snack
	Main Course
Type of Dish	Vegetarian
	Non-Vegetarian
Preparation Time	Approximately 10 minutes
	Approximately 10 minutes, baking time
	Approximately 30 minutes, soaking time
Cooking Time	Approximately 10 minutes
Servings	4
The AilamA® Cookbook advises You	You can bake raw buckwheat with salt in the oven for 5 minutes for a nutty taste. Serve it instead of popcorn when watching a good movie.

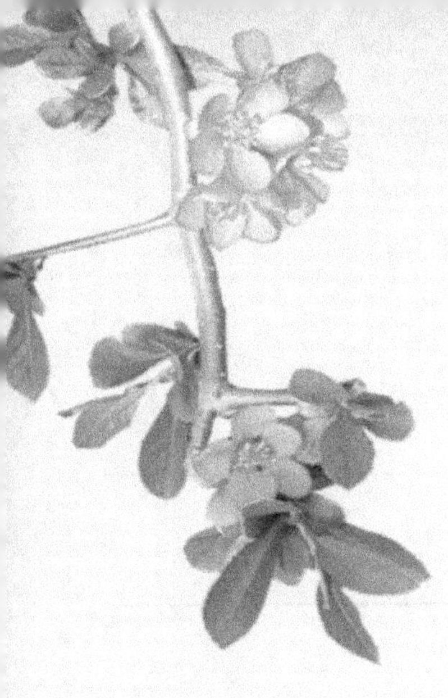

INGREDIENTS

1 handful buckwheat, previously soaked in water for 30 minutes
1 bunch baby spinach *or* valerian *or* arugula
1 sweet red pepper, moderately diced
1 onion, moderately diced, previously baked
2 tablespoons extra virgin olive oil
½ lemon, juiced
¼ teaspoon unrefined sea salt

PREPARATION

1. Boil buckwheat for 10 minutes. *(See also pages 48, 61, and 152.)*
2. Let buckwheat cool.
3. Put baby spinach in a glass bowl.
4. Add buckwheat, pepper, oil, lemon, salt.
5. Mix well.
6. Serve as a side dish or by itself.

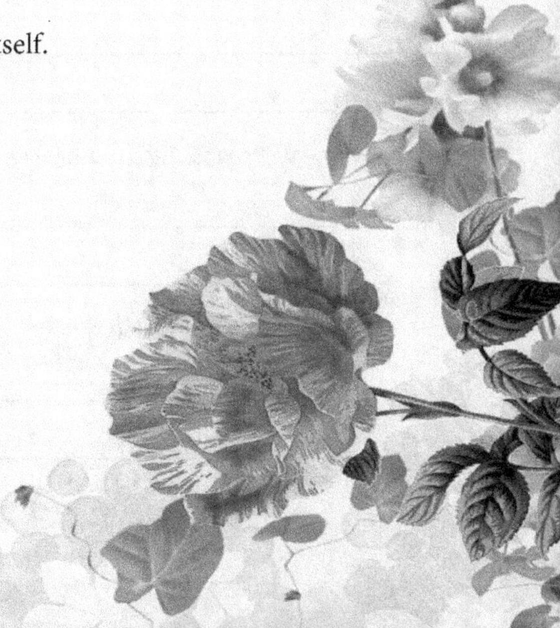

You Matter!

1. Take four gorgeous pictures of your culinary result.

2. Write down your impressions of the recipe.

a. Did you like it?

____

b. Was it difficult?

____

c. Did you find all the ingredients?

____

d. Did you make any changes to the recipe to better suit your dietary needs?

____

____

e. Will you cook it again?

____

f. Will you share it with your family and friends?

____

g. How did it make your body feel?

____

____

h. How were you feeling before cooking the recipe?

____

____

i. How were you feeling after eating the culinary result?

____

____

HOMEMADE MOZZARELLA

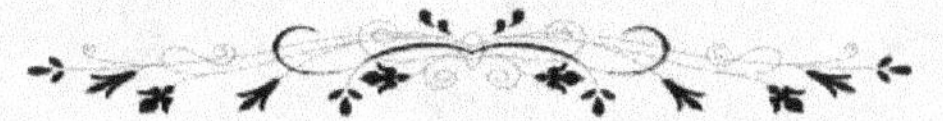

Here is the recipe for a very special type of cheese.

Whether you choose to eat it as it is or in different combinations, you will absolutely adore it, guaranteed !

You can also enjoy it when you feel deeply satisfied with what you've got.

Type of Meal	Snack Appetizer
Type of Dish	Lacto-Vegetarian Non-Vegetarian
Preparation Time	Approximately 5 minutes
Cooking Time	Approximately 30 minutes
Servings	10
The AilamA® Cookbook advises You	You can use it as a healthy ingredient in homemade pizza. *(See also page 231.)* You can adjust the amount of salt to your own taste. If you want your cheese to have a softer, elastic consistency, don't strain all the whey from it.

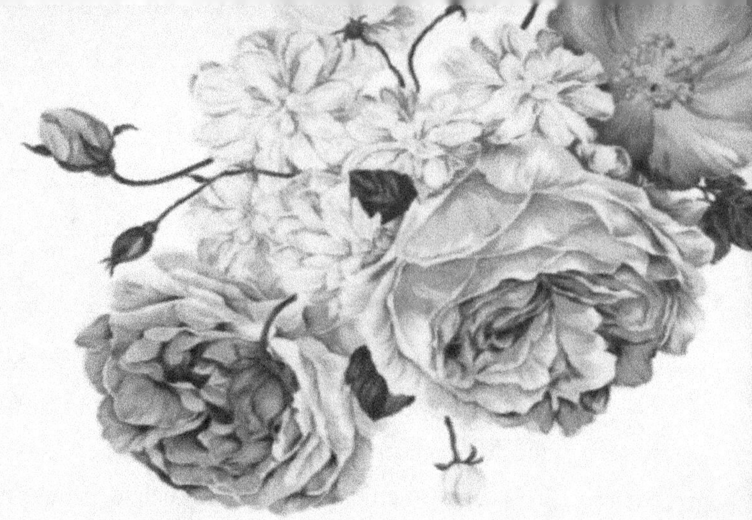

INGREDIENTS

2 liters (~70 fl oz) skim milk *(organic)*
or
2 liters (~70 fl oz) whole milk *(bio)*
1 teaspoonful unrefined rock salt
½ teaspoonful fresh lemon juice

PREPARATION

1. Let milk sit at room temperature overnight.
2. Add lemon juice to milk.
3. Bring milk to a boil, until curds separate from whey.
4. Don't let milk boil.
5. Strain curdled milk.
6. Add salt and mix well with wooden spoon.
7. Leave curdled milk in strain, until no more whey comes out.
8. Keep it in the refrigerator.
9. Serve cold, chilled, or at room temperature.

You Matter!

1. Take four gorgeous pictures of your culinary result.

2. Write down your impressions of the recipe.

a. Did you like it?

____

b. Was it difficult?

____

c. Did you find all the ingredients?

____

d. Did you make any changes to the recipe to better suit your dietary needs?

____

____

e. Will you cook it again?

____

f. Will you share it with your family and friends?

____

g. How did it make your body feel?

____

____

h. How were you feeling before cooking the recipe?

____

____

i. How were you feeling after eating the culinary result?

____

____

ALMOND CAKE

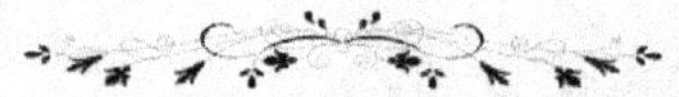

Here is yet another dish prepared with healthy ingredients for you and your family. This flour-free cake is also perfect to satisfy your daily craving for sweets, regardless of your emotional state.

Type of Meal	Snack
	Dessert
Type of Dish	Lacto-Ovo-Vegetarian
	Non-Vegetarian
Preparation Time	Approximately 10 minutes
	Approximately 30 minutes, refrigeration time
Cooking Time	Approximately 30 minutes
Servings	16 pieces
The AilamA® Cookbook advises You	You can replace almonds with walnuts, if you like.

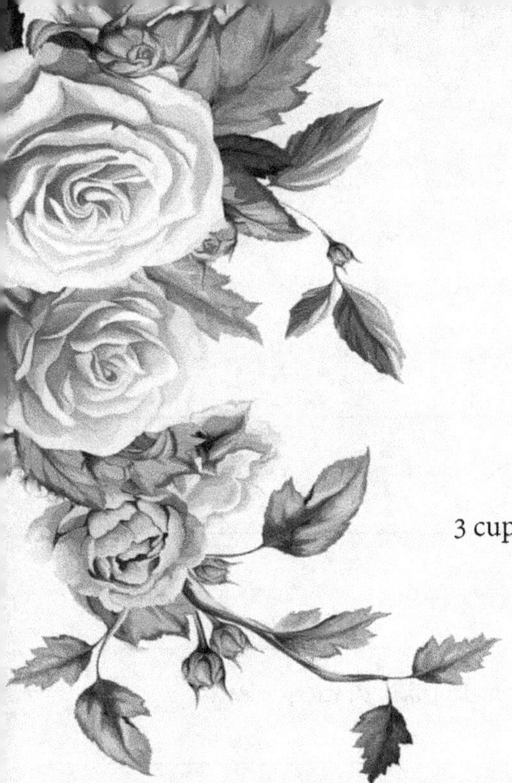

INGREDIENTS

1 large egg
½ pack (clarified) butter
½ small cup coconut blossom sugar
½ teaspoon pure vanilla extract
½ small cup natural plum jam
½ teaspoon carob powder
3 cups (germinated) almonds *or* walnuts, coarsely ground
Cooking spray *(coconut oil)*
Pinch of natural salt

PREPARATION

1. Preheat oven to 160 degrees C (320 degrees F).
2. Put butter, sugar, egg, and vanilla in blender.
3. Mix ingredients until light and fluffy.
4. Add almonds, carob powder, and salt.
5. Whisk until well combined.
6. Refrigerate batter for 30 minutes.
7. Spread it on a baking sheet, lightly coated with cooking spray.
8. Spread plum jam on top.
9. Bake for about 20 minutes.
10. Remove from oven.
11. Cut when cold.
12. Serve at room temperature.

You Matter!

1. Take four gorgeous pictures of your culinary result.

2. Write down your impressions of the recipe.

a. Did you like it?

____

b. Was it difficult?

____

c. Did you find all the ingredients?

____

d. Did you make any changes to the recipe to better suit your dietary needs?

____

____

e. Will you cook it again?

____

f. Will you share it with your family and friends?

____

g. How did it make your body feel?

____

____

h. How were you feeling before cooking the recipe?

____

____

i. How were you feeling after eating the culinary result?

____

____

HAPPY OILS

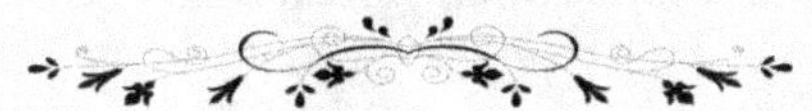

You can practically make happy oils out of lots of dried or seedy ingredients. Here are some tips.

Type of Recipe	Cosmetic Ingredient
Category of People	Vegetarians Non-Vegetarians
Preparation Time	Approximately 2 minutes
Macerating Time	Approximately 1 month
Servings	Approximately 200 ml (6.8 fl oz)
The AilamA® Cookbook advises You	Happy oils can be used by themselves or in cosmetic creams, lotions, and scrubs. You can combine any of the ingredients listed below with a mild-flavored oil of your choice.

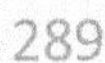

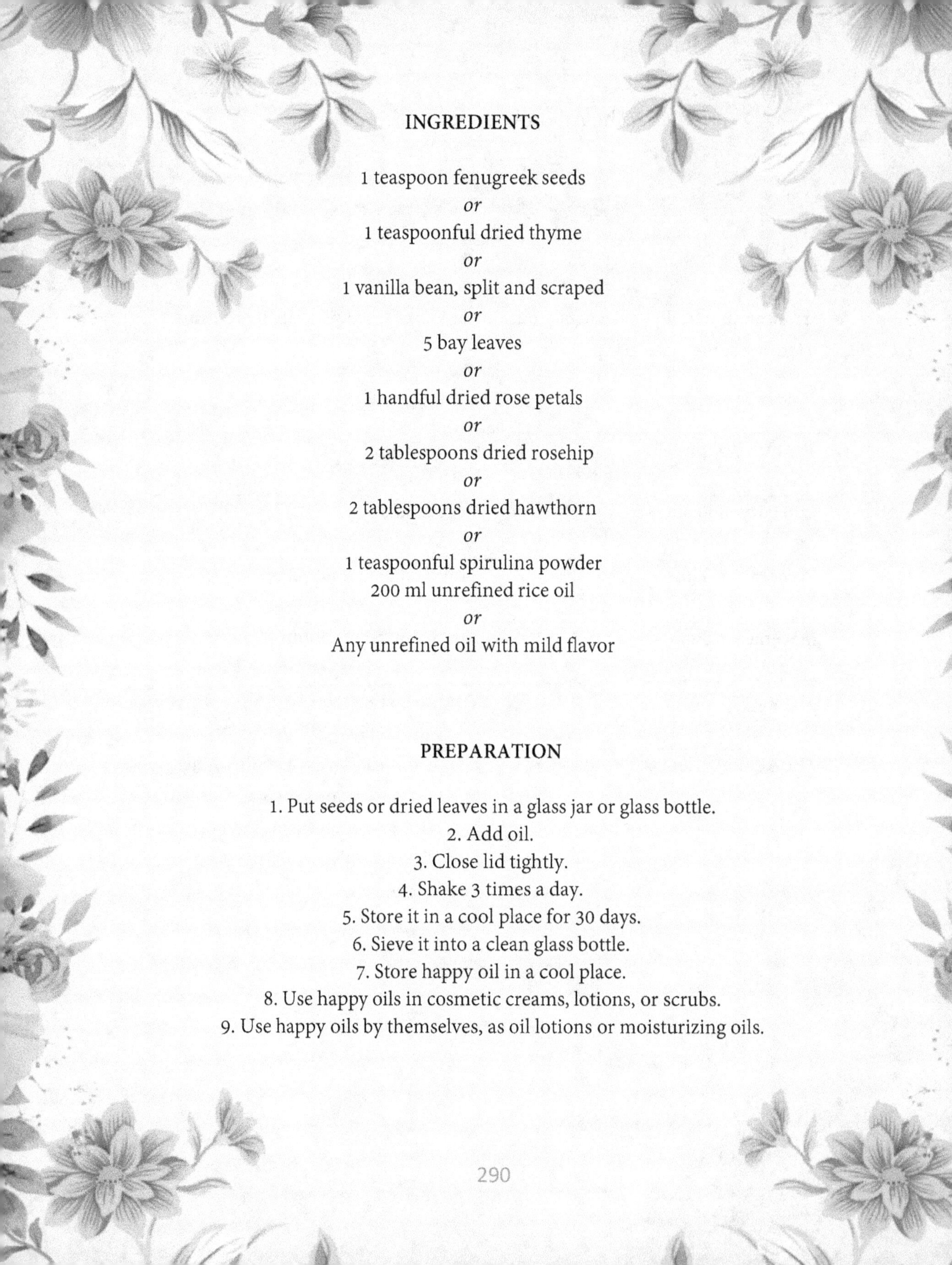

INGREDIENTS

1 teaspoon fenugreek seeds

or

1 teaspoonful dried thyme

or

1 vanilla bean, split and scraped

or

5 bay leaves

or

1 handful dried rose petals

or

2 tablespoons dried rosehip

or

2 tablespoons dried hawthorn

or

1 teaspoonful spirulina powder

200 ml unrefined rice oil

or

Any unrefined oil with mild flavor

PREPARATION

1. Put seeds or dried leaves in a glass jar or glass bottle.
2. Add oil.
3. Close lid tightly.
4. Shake 3 times a day.
5. Store it in a cool place for 30 days.
6. Sieve it into a clean glass bottle.
7. Store happy oil in a cool place.
8. Use happy oils in cosmetic creams, lotions, or scrubs.
9. Use happy oils by themselves, as oil lotions or moisturizing oils.

You Matter!

1. Take four gorgeous pictures of your result.

2. Write down your impressions of the recipe.

a. What are you going to do with your Happy Oil?

____

b. Was it a difficult recipe?

____

c. Did you find all of the ingredients?

____

d. Did you make any changes to the recipe to better suit your personal taste?

____

____

e. Will you try the recipe again?

____

f. Will you share the recipe with your family and friends?

____

g. How did your Happy Oil make your skin feel?

____

____

h. How were you feeling before trying the recipe?

____

____

i. How were you feeling after trying the result?

____

____

The AilamA® Special Recipe 2

HAPPY HAIR

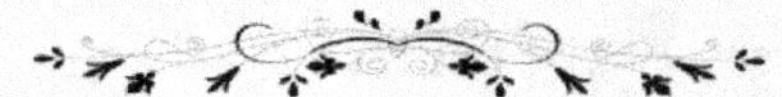

Did you know that you could go no poo? This actually means that you can stop using regular shampoo and conditioner.

Try this hair recipe for yourself and see what happens.

Type of Recipe	Beauty Hack
Category of People	Vegetarians Non-Vegetarians
Preparation Time	Approximately 2 minutes
Washing Time	Approximately 10 minutes
Servings	1 hair wash
The AilamA® Cookbook advises You	If your hair is short, you can use less baking soda and vinegar. You needn't apply baking soda from the roots to the ends. All of your hair will get properly washed when you rinse off your scalp, from the baking soda dissolved in the water running down your locks.

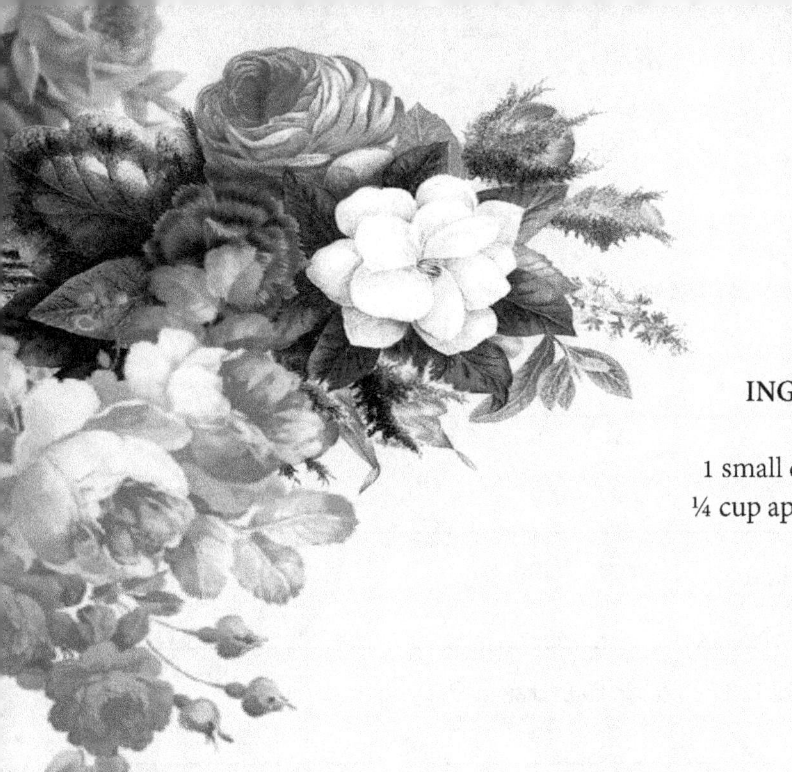

INGREDIENTS

1 small cup baking soda
¼ cup apple cider vinegar

INSTRUCTIONS

1. Wet your hair.
2. Take as much baking soda as you can between your fingertips.
3. Rub it into the roots of your hair, all over the scalp.
4. Rub and massage your scalp well.
5. Rinse thoroughly.
6. Repeat procedure.
7. Rinse thoroughly.
8. Combine apple cider vinegar with warm water in a pot on hand.
9. Rinse hair with the vinegar solution.
10. Massage the solution into your scalp and on your hair's length.
11. Rinse thoroughly with water.
12. Wash your hair once a week.

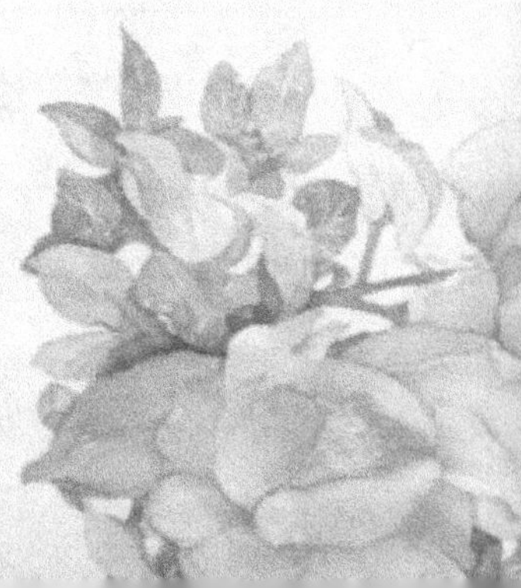

You Matter!

1. Take four gorgeous selfies after you have tried the Happy Hair recipe.

2. Write down your impressions of the recipe.

a. Did you like it?

____

b. Was it difficult?

____

c. Did you find all the ingredients?

____

d. Did you make any changes to the recipe to better suit your hair type?

____

____

e. Will you try the recipe again?

____

f. Will you share the recipe with your family and friends?

____

g. What did your hair look and feel like after trying this washing method?

____

____

h. How were you feeling before trying this washing method?

____

____

i. How were you feeling after trying this washing method?

____

____

AilamA®

EMOTIONAL

NUTRITION PROGRAM

A 28-Day Eating Program for You and Your Family

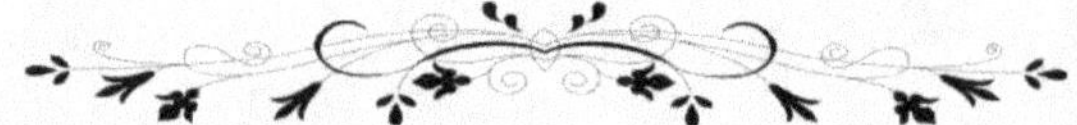

It's true, we come in different body shapes that have different genetic predispositions. Yet we don't really have to be experts in science in order to understand our own bodies.

What if we don't take much pleasure in counting our daily caloric intake, but still want to get the perfect body size that promotes optimal health?

Yes, we can achieve that by understanding our dietary needs based on our genetic inheritance as well as our life habits.

However, we may find it tiring to always count how much protein, carbohydrate, or fat is in each meal. Moreover, this regular counting may rob us of our instinctual guidelines, the true voice of our individualities.

The rest does come down to statistics and figures.

The AilamA® Nutrition Program is a 28-day meal plan that respects the general nutrition guidelines we can find in any reliable specialty book, without focusing on endless calculations of calories or on exact percentages of healthy nutrients such as proteins, carbohydrates, fats, vitamins, and minerals.

Unless you are in desperate need of a dramatic dietary change on grounds of poor health, in which case you should consult a local professional, The AilamA® Nutrition Program can provide you with a different view on your eating routines. Moreover, it can help you embrace your emotional eating and accept, once and for all, that you will always feel certain emotions before, while, and after eating.

As to the basic nutrition information, you can find it with one mouse click, or several, in any cyber-reality connected to this field of interest.

It is your personalized nutrition guide that can't just be computed out of general facts. An accurate diet calculator can only follow your trustworthy instincts, thus translating knowledge into action.

You can be your own nutritionist! You can create a unique eating program based on your personal principles of staying healthy.

However, if you find it difficult to lose weight and change your dietary habits by yourself, feel free to consult a certified nutritionist to get all the help you need along the way.

Always listen to your own body!

DAY ONE

BREAKFAST
1 **Alga Frittata** (*Week 1, page 11*)
2 slices of **Bread Booster** (*Week 11, page 63*)
MORNING SNACK
1 moderate bowl of **Butter Fruit Cocktail** (*Week 17, page 104*)
LUNCH
1 moderate bowl of **Millet Pudding** (*Week 8, page 47*)
AFTERNOON SNACK
8 **Patties** (*Week 14, page 81*)
DINNER
6 pieces of **Big Sushi** (*Week 10, page 59*)
2 teaspoons of **Pickled Horseradish** (*Week 10, page 56*)

DAY TWO

BREAKFAST
1 slice of **Bread Booster** (*Week 11, page 63*)
1 tablespoon of organic butter
MORNING SNACK
4 pieces of **Veg-Sushi** (*Week 15, page 92*)
LUNCH
1 moderate plate of **Royal Wok** (*Week 4, page 28*)
2 palm-sized slices of **Baked Beef** (*Week 24, page 134*)
AFTERNOON SNACK
4 pieces of **Fluffy Cake** (*Week 11, page 66*)
DINNER
1 moderate bowl of **Smartly Dressed Salad** (*Week 6, page 41*)
2 palm-sized slices of broiled turkey breast

DAY THREE

BREAKFAST
1 moderate bowl of **Cranberry Salad** *(Week 9, page 53)*
MORNING SNACK
4 pieces of **O-Sushi** *(Week 26, page 149)*
LUNCH
1 moderate bowl of **Meaty Soup** *(Week 7, page 44)*
1 slice of **Bread Booster** *(Week 11, page 63)*
AFTERNOON SNACK
3 pieces of **Choco Cake** *(Week 15, page 88)*
DINNER
1 moderate bowl of **Parsley Salad** *(Week 13, page 75)*
1 **Cocktail Skewer** *(Week 16, page 98)*

DAY FOUR

BREAKFAST
5 pieces of **Berry Cake** *(Week 16, page 95)*
MORNING SNACK
2 slices of **Bread Booster** *(Week 11, page 63)*
2 slices of **Homemade Pressed Cheese** *(Week 5, page 35)*
LUNCH
1 moderate plate of **Bean Noodles Yum** *(Week 2, page 17)*
AFTERNOON SNACK
1 small pot of **Choco-Nut** *(Week 12, page 69)*
4 tablespoons of **Homemade Yogurt** *(Week 12, page 72)*
DINNER
1 moderate bowl of **Sweet-Sour Chicken** *(Week 18, page 107)*

DAY FIVE

BREAKFAST
4 **Whey Pancakes** *(Week 5, page 38)*
1 cup of **Milk Thistle Crunch** *(Week 14, page 85)*
MORNING SNACK
2 tablespoons of **Homemade Pâté** *(Week 17, page 101)*
1 slice of **Bread Booster** *(Week 11, page 63)*
LUNCH
1 moderate bowl of **Seaweed Salad** *(Week 25, page 140)*
2 palm-sized slices of **Baked Beef** *(Week 24, page 134)*
AFTERNOON SNACK
6 tablespoons of **Tuna Dipping Sauce** *(Week 1, page 14)*
4 moderate slices of sweet pointed red pepper
DINNER
1 moderate bowl of **Broccoli Wok** *(Week 20, page 146)*

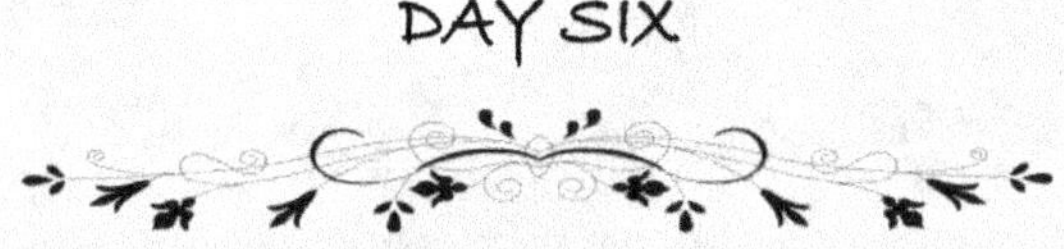

DAY SIX

BREAKFAST
1 slice of **Bread Booster** *(Week 11, page 63)*
1 cup of **Homemade Kefir** *(Week 3, page 25)*
MORNING SNACK
1 moderate cup of **Fig Truffles** *(Week 13, page 78)*
LUNCH
1 moderate plate of **Quinoa Wok Veggie** *(Week 3, page 21)*
1 palm-sized slice of broiled turkey thigh, skinless and boneless
AFTERNOON SNACK
1 small pot of **Choco-Delight** *(Week 23, page 128)*
DINNER
1 moderate bowl of **Potato & Mushroom Stew** *(Week 22, page 125)*

DAY SEVEN

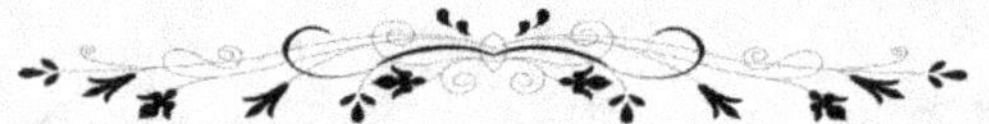

BREAKFAST
2 moderate slices of **Homemade Pressed Cheese** *(Week 5, page 35)*
½ iceberg salad with **Cheddar Nut Dressing** *(Week 24, page 137)*
MORNING SNACK
1 small pot of **Minty Brown Cream** *(Week 22, page 122)*
LUNCH
1 moderate plate of **Veggie Stew** *(Week 23, page 131)*
AFTERNOON SNACK
1 small pot of **Choco-Exotique** *(Week 26, page 146)*
DINNER
1 moderate plate of **Leek Wok** *(Week 19, page 113)*

DAY EIGHT

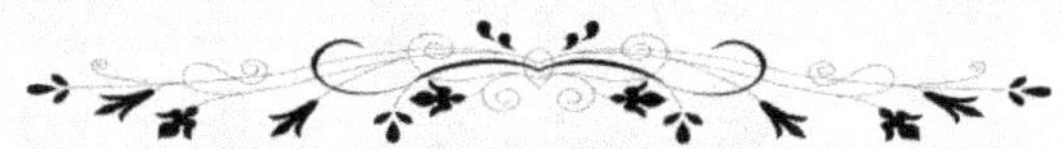

BREAKFAST
2 slices of **Pizza Chameleon** *(Week 41, page 231)*
MORNING SNACK
1 moderate bowl of **Salmon-Chicken Salad** *(Week 48, page 263)*
LUNCH
1 moderate bowl of **Rice Boost** *(Week 27, page 152)*
AFTERNOON SNACK
8 **Chicory Sweet-Eyed Cookies** *(Week 31, page 180)*
DINNER
6 pieces of **Old Sushi** *(Week 29, page 165)*
2 **Pickled Cucumbers** *(Week 34, page 198)*

DAY NINE

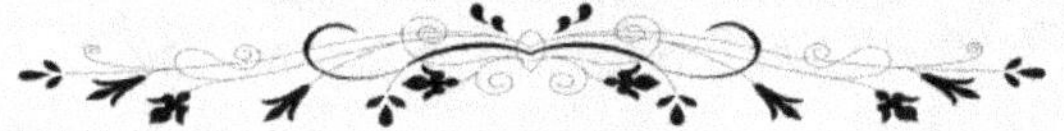

BREAKFAST
3 **Dinkel Flatties** *(Week 30, page 171)*
3 slices of **Kefir Cheese** *(Week 38, page 216)*
MORNING SNACK
4 pieces of **T-Sushi** *(Week 46, page 256)*
LUNCH
1 moderate plate of **Cheerful Wok** *(Week 34, page 195)*
4 meatballs of **Minced Mix** *(Week 43, page 241)*
AFTERNOON SNACK
¼ **Baked Squash** *(Week 28, page 162)*
DINNER
1 moderate bowl of **Sweet Potato Salad** *(Week 36, page 207)*
2 palm-sized slices of broiled chicken breast

DAY TEN

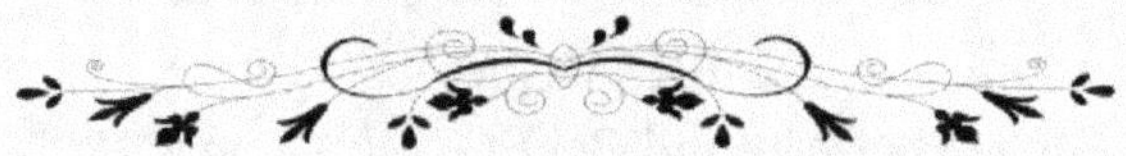

BREAKFAST
1 moderate bowl of **Mixed Salad** *(Week 40, page 228)*
MORNING SNACK
½ **Baked Quince** *(Week 29, page 168)*
LUNCH
1 moderate bowl of **Veggie White Delight** *(Week 28, page 158)*
AFTERNOON SNACK
3 pieces of **Sweet-Sour Comfy** *(Week 30, page 174)*
DINNER
1 moderate bowl of **Broil & Bake Salad** *(Week 33, page 189)*
2 broiled chicken thighs, skinless and boneless

DAY ELEVEN

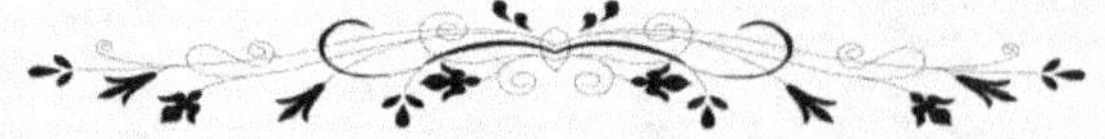

BREAKFAST
5 pieces of **Raspberry Cake** (*Week 39, page 225*)
MORNING SNACK
2 slices of **Dinkel Flatties** (*Week 30, page 171*)
2 slices of **Homemade Mozzarella** (*Week 52, page 283*)
LUNCH
1 moderate bowl of **Veggie Cream** (*Week 47, page 259*)
AFTERNOON SNACK
1 small pot of **Caramel Pudding** (*Week 33, page 192*)
1 small cup of **Chico-Tea** (*Week 41, page 235*)
DINNER
1 moderate bowl of **Stir Fried Eggplants** (*Week 35, page 201*)

DAY TWELVE

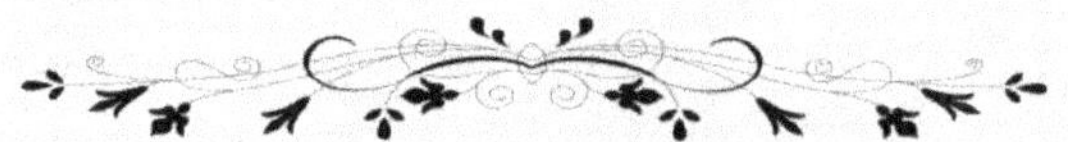

BREAKFAST
4 pieces of **Almond Cake** (*Week 52, page 286*)
1 small cup of **Dandelion-Root Coffee** (*Week 45, page 253*)
MORNING SNACK
6 **Truffles Chameleon** (*Week 18, page 110*)
LUNCH
1 moderate plate of **Wok Delight** (*Week 39, page 222*)
1 palm-sized slice of broiled turkey thigh, skinless and boneless
AFTERNOON SNACK
1 small pot of **Caro-Cream** (*Week 8, page 50*)
1 small bowl of no-salt, oil-free popcorn
DINNER
1 moderate bowl of **Thy Stew** (*Week 49, page 273*)

DAY THIRTEEN

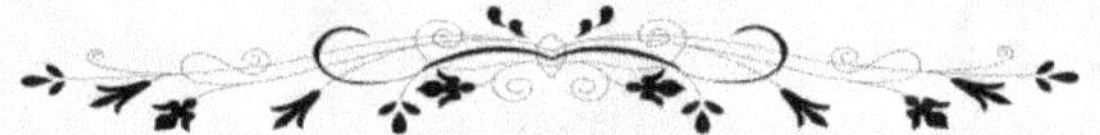

BREAKFAST
8 pieces of **Cinnamon Spice Sweet** *(Week 35, page 204)*
1 cup of **Caro-Coffee** *(Week 4, page 32)*
MORNING SNACK
3 tablespoons of **Mashed Black Bean** *(Week 31, page 177)*
1 slice of **Bread Booster** *(Week 11, page 63)*
LUNCH
1 moderate bowl of **Buckwheat Salad** *(Week 51, page 280)*
2 palm-sized slices of **Baked Beef** *(Week 24, page 134)*
AFTERNOON SNACK
2 tablespoons of **Mashed Parsnips** *(Week 50, page 277)*
1moderate slice of **Kefir Cheese** *(Week 38, page 216)*
DINNER
1 moderate bowl of **Cabbage Wok** *(Week 37, page 213)*

DAY FOURTEEN

BREAKFAST
½ iceberg salad with **Red Pepper Dipping Sauce** *(Week 44, page 247)*
4 pieces of **Squash Cake** *(Week 36, page 210)*
MORNING SNACK
1 slice of **Chocolate Sweet Delight** *(Week 48, page 266)*
LUNCH
1 moderate plate of **Macrobiotic Soup** *(Week 42, page 238)*
AFTERNOON SNACK
5 pieces of **Cinnamon Spice Sweet** *(Week 35, page 204)*
DINNER
1 moderate plate of **Brocco White Delight** *(Week 32, page 183)*

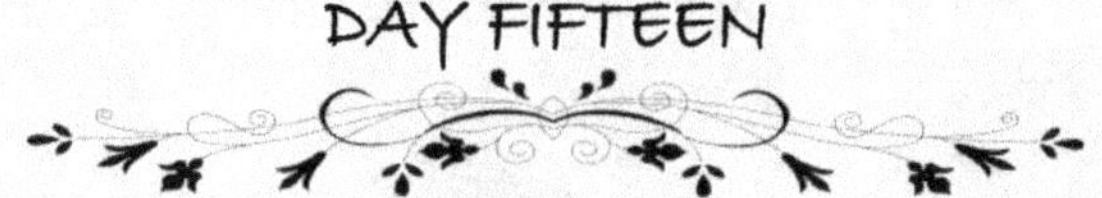

DAY FIFTEEN

BREAKFAST
4 **Whey Pancakes** *(Week 5, page 38)*
1 cup of **Caro-Coffee** *(Week 4, page 32)*
MORNING SNACK
2 tablespoons of **Ruby Sour-Sweet** *(Week 25, page 143)*
1 slice of **Bread Booster** *(Week 11, page 63)*
LUNCH
1 moderate plate of **Quinoa Wok Veggie** *(Week 3, page 21)*
1 palm-sized slice of broiled chicken thigh, skinless and boneless
AFTERNOON SNACK
3 tablespoons of **Mashed Parsnips** *(Week 50, page 277)*
2 moderate slices of sweet pointed red pepper
DINNER
1 moderate bowl of **China Mix** *(Week 21, page 119)*

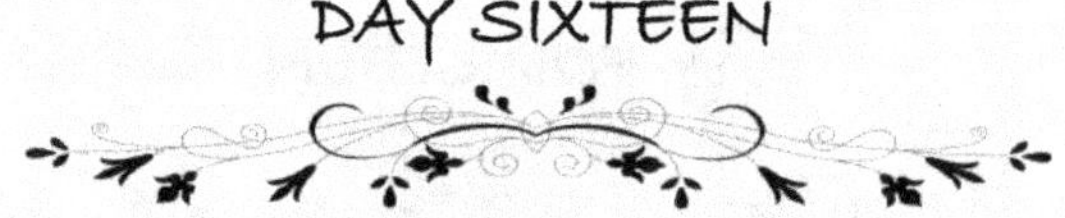

DAY SIXTEEN

BREAKFAST
6 pieces of **K-Sushi** *(Week 38, page 219)*
MORNING SNACK
½ small cup of **Honey-Delight** *(Week 27, page 155)*
LUNCH
1 moderate bowl of **Sweet Potato Salad** *(Week 36, page 207)*
AFTERNOON SNACK
1 slice of **Pizza Chameleon** *(Week 41, page 231)*
DINNER
1 moderate bowl of **Potato & Mushroom Stew** *(Week 22, page 125)*

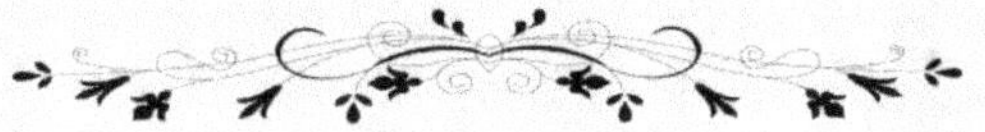

DAY SEVENTEEN

BREAKFAST
2 moderate slices of **Homemade Pressed Cheese** *(Week 5, page 35)*
1 slice of **Bread Booster** *(Week 11, page 63)*
2 tablespoons of **Plum Yum-Yum** *(Week 32, page 186)*
MORNING SNACK
8 **Chicory Sweet-Eyed Cookies** *(Week 31, page 180)*
LUNCH
1 moderate bowl of **Rice Boost** *(Week 27, page 152)*
AFTERNOON SNACK
6 pieces of **Old Sushi** *(Week 29, page 165)*
DINNER
1 moderate bowl of **Salmon-Chicken Salad** *(Week 48, page 263)*

DAY EIGHTEEN

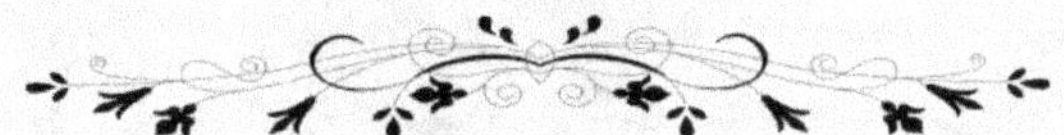

BREAKFAST
2 slices of **Pizza Chameleon** *(Week 41, page 231)*
MORNING SNACK
4 pieces of **Prune Cake** *(Week 45, page 250)*
LUNCH
1 moderate bowl of **Seaweed Salad** *(Week 25, page 140)*
2 palm-sized slices of **Baked Beef** *(Week 24, page 134)*
AFTERNOON SNACK
2 tablespoons of **Homemade Pâté** *(Week 17, page 101)*
1 slice of **Bread Booster** *(Week 11, page 63)*
DINNER
1 small bowl of **Potato & Mushroom Stew** *(Week 22, page 125)*

DAY NINETEEN

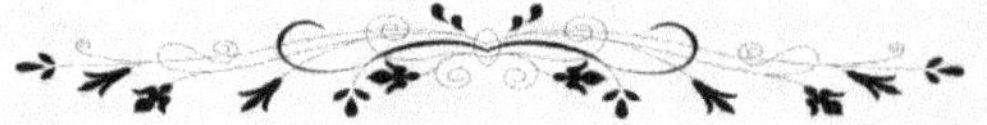

BREAKFAST
3 **Dinkel Flatties** *(Week 30, page 171)*
3 slices of **Kefir Cheese** *(Week 38, page 216)*
MORNING SNACK
4 pieces of **T-Sushi** *(Week 46, page 256)*
LUNCH
1 moderate plate of **Cheerful Wok** *(Week 34, page 195)*
4 meatballs of **Minced Mix** *(Week 43, page 241)*
AFTERNOON SNACK
2 **Baked Apples** *(Week 43, page 244)*
DINNER
1 moderate bowl of **Sweet Potato Salad** *(Week 36, page 207)*
2 palm-sized slices of broiled chicken breast

DAY TWENTY

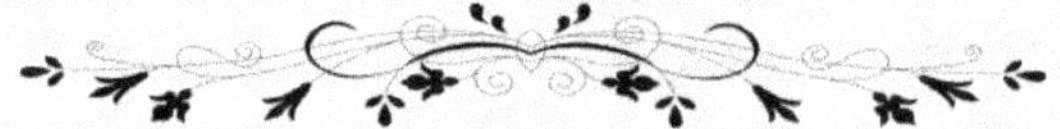

BREAKFAST
1 moderate bowl of **Cranberry Salad** *(Week 9, page 53)*
MORNING SNACK
4 pieces of **O-Sushi** *(Week 26, page 149)*
LUNCH
1 moderate bowl of **Meaty Soup** *(Week 7, page 44)*
1 slice of **Bread Booster** *(Week 11, page 63)*
AFTERNOON SNACK
3 pieces of **Coco Cold** *(Week 49, page 270)*
DINNER
1 moderate bowl of **Parsley Salad** *(Week 13, page 75)*
1 **Cocktail Skewer** *(Week 16, page 98)*

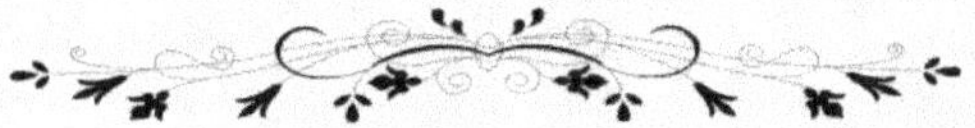

DAY TWENTY-ONE

BREAKFAST
8 pieces of **Cinnamon Spice Sweet** *(Week 35, page 204)*
2 tablespoons of **Homemade Yogurt** *(Week 12, page 72)*
MORNING SNACK
1 slice of **Homemade Mozzarella** *(Week 52, page 283)*
1 slice of **Bread Booster** *(Week 11, page 63)*
LUNCH
1 moderate bowl of **Buckwheat Salad** *(Week 51, page 280)*
2 palm-sized slices of **Baked Beef** *(Week 24, page 134)*
AFTERNOON SNACK
2 tablespoons of **Mashed Parsnips** *(Week 50, page 277)*
1 slice of **Bread Booster** *(Week 11, page 63)*
DINNER
1 moderate bowl of **Stir Fried Eggplants** *(Week 35, page 201)*

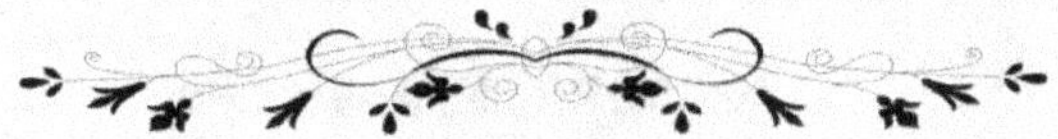

DAY TWENTY-TWO

BREAKFAST
1 **Alga Frittata** *(Week 1, page 11)*
2 slices of **Bread Booster** *(Week 11, page 63)*
MORNING SNACK
1 moderate bowl of **Butter Fruit Cocktail** *(Week 17, page 104)*
LUNCH
1 moderate bowl of **Rice Boost** *(Week 27, page 152)*
AFTERNOON SNACK
8 **Patties** *(Week 14, page 81)*
DINNER
6 pieces of **O-Sushi** *(Week 26, page 149)*
2 teaspoons of **Pickled Horseradish** *(Week 10, page 56)*

DAY TWENTY-THREE

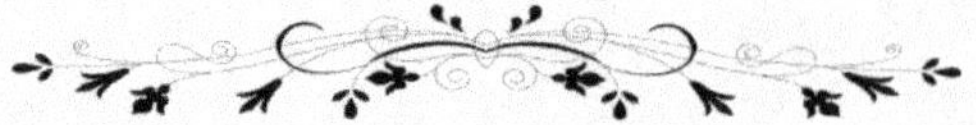

BREAKFAST
5 pieces of **Raspberry Cake** *(Week 39, page 225)*
MORNING SNACK
2 slices of **Dinkel Flatties** *(Week 30, page 171)*
2 slices of **Homemade Pâté** *(Week 17, page 101)*
LUNCH
1 moderate bowl of **Veggie Stew** *(Week 23, page 131)*
AFTERNOON SNACK
1 small pot of **Caramel Pudding** *(Week 33, page 192)*
DINNER
1 moderate bowl of **China Mix** *(Week 21, page 119)*

DAY TWENTY-FOUR

BREAKFAST
4 **Whey Pancakes** *(Week 5, page 38)*
1 cup of **Dandelion-Root Coffee** *(Week 45, page 253)*
MORNING SNACK
2 tablespoons of **Homemade Pâté** *(Week 17, page 101)*
1 slice of **Bread Booster** *(Week 11, page 63)*
LUNCH
1 moderate bowl of **Salmon-Chicken Salad** *(Week 48, page 263)*
AFTERNOON SNACK
6 tablespoons of **Tuna Dipping Sauce** *(Week 1, page 14)*
4 moderate slices of sweet pointed red pepper
DINNER
1 moderate bowl of **Broccoli Wok** *(Week 20, page 146)*

DAY TWENTY-FIVE

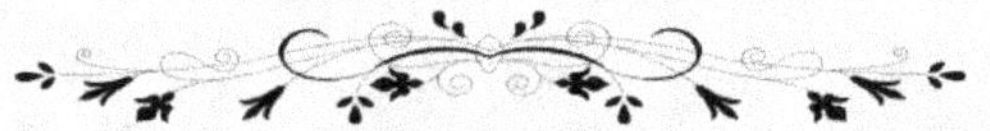

BREAKFAST
1 slice of **Bread Booster** *(Week 11, page 63)*
1 tablespoon of clarified butter
MORNING SNACK
4 pieces of **Veg-Sushi** *(Week 15, page 92)*
LUNCH
1 moderate plate of **Royal Wok** *(Week 4, page 28)*
AFTERNOON SNACK
4 pieces of **Fluffy Cake** *(Week 11, page 66)*
DINNER
1 moderate bowl of **Thy Stew** *(Week 49, page 273)*

DAY TWENTY-SIX

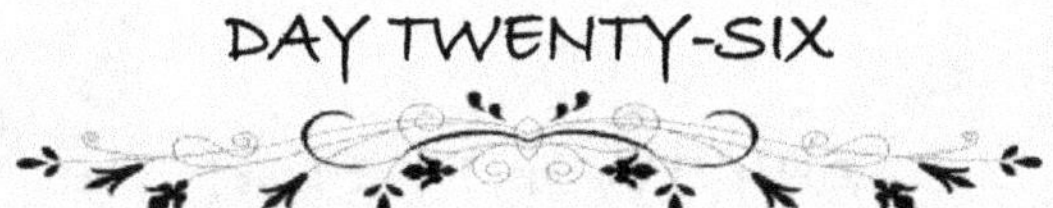

BREAKFAST
4 pieces of **Almond Cake** *(Week 52, page 286)*
1 small cup of **Caro-Coffee** *(Week 4, page 32)*
MORNING SNACK
6 **Truffles Chameleon** *(Week 18, page 110)*
LUNCH
1 moderate plate of **Royal Wok** *(Week 4, page 28)*
1 palm-sized slice of broiled chicken thigh, skinless and boneless
AFTERNOON SNACK
1 small pot of **Caro-Cream** *(Week 8, page 50)*
1 small bowl of no-salt, oil-free popcorn
DINNER
1 moderate bowl of **Thy Stew** *(Week 49, page 273)*

DAY TWENTY-SEVEN

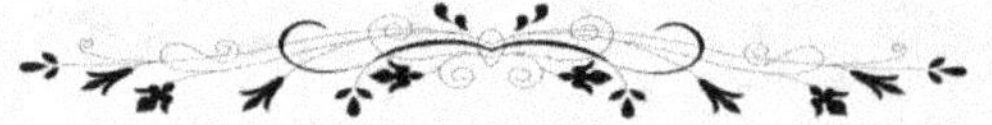

BREAKFAST
2 moderate slices of **Homemade Pressed Cheese** *(Week 5, page 35)*
1 slice of **Bread Booster** *(Week 11, page 63)*
MORNING SNACK
8 **Chicory Sweet-Eyed Cookies** *(Week 31, page 180)*
LUNCH
1 moderate bowl of **Millet Pudding** *(Week 8, page 47)*
AFTERNOON SNACK
6 pieces of **Old Sushi** *(Week 29, page 165)*
DINNER
1 moderate bowl of **Bean Noodles Yum** *(Week 2, page 17)*

DAY TWENTY-EIGHT

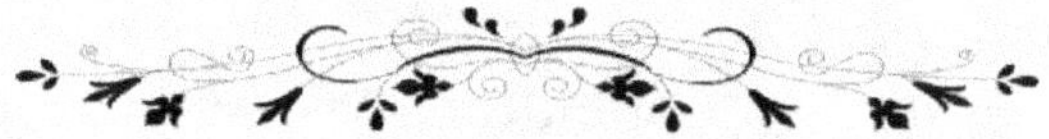

BREAKFAST
1 moderate bowl of **Sweet Potato Salad** *(Week 36, page 207)*
MORNING SNACK
2 **Baked Apples** *(Week 43, page 244)*
LUNCH
3 slices of **Pizza Chameleon** *(Week 41, page 231)*
AFTERNOON SNACK
8 **Patties** *(Week 14, page 81)*
DINNER
1 moderate bowl of **China Mix** *(Week 21, page 119)*

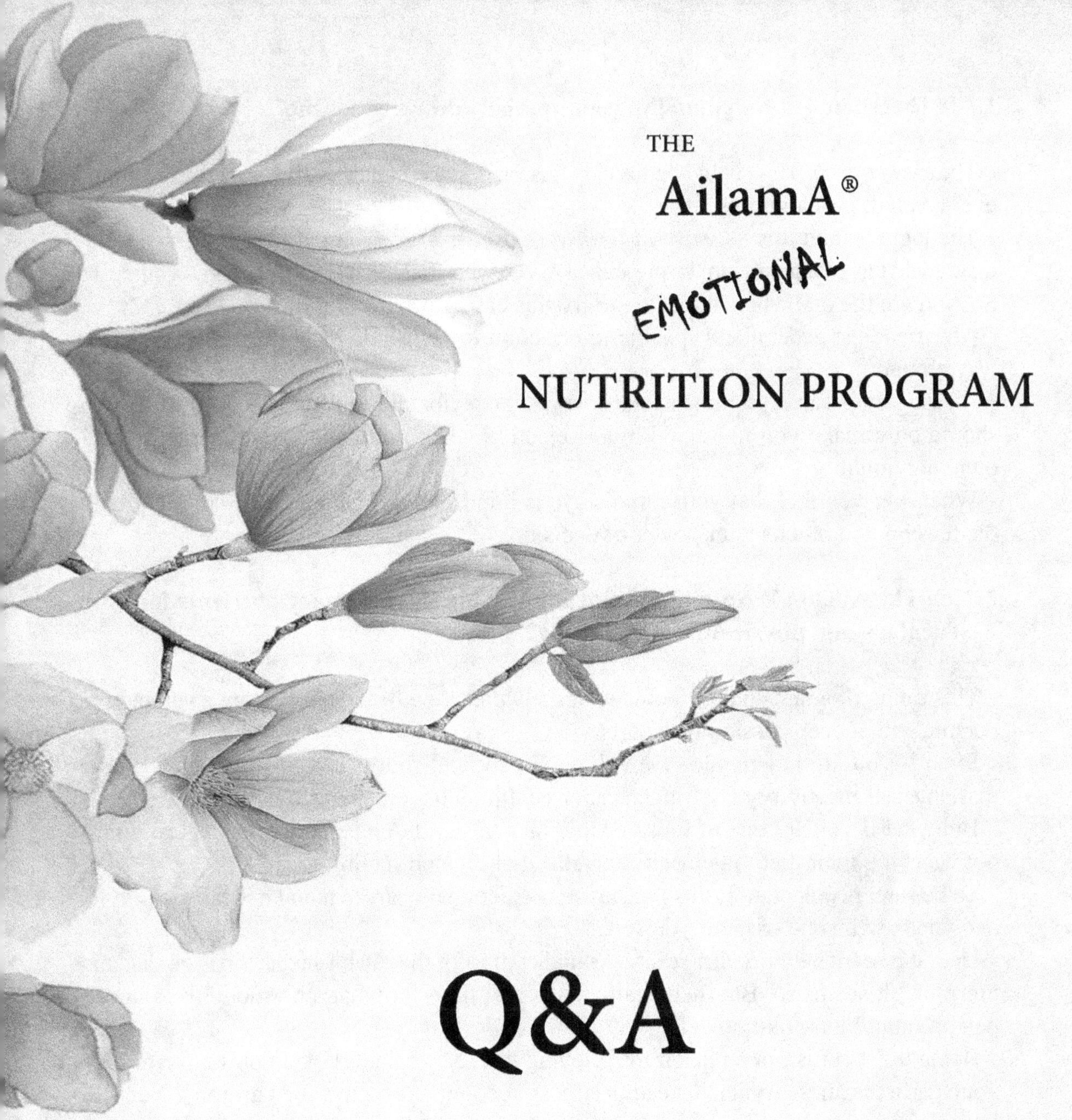

Here are some guiding questions, whose answers you should read carefully before embarking on your own dietary journey, inspired by The AilamA® Nutrition Program.

1. Is The AilamA® Nutrition Program specially designed for me?

The answer is *no*. This should be the only answer when it comes to all nutritional programs ever created, past and present.

The logic behind this *negative-in-form* yet *positive-in-meaning* answer is very simple: How could this eating program be prescribed to you when only you are able to know yourself? So, you are the one who can decide to try this eating program or not.

Always adjust general and specific information to your individual needs, not the other way around.

All suggestions and recommendations for attaining vibrant health and personal wellbeing should only make you more and more selective when you have taken charge of your own individuality.

Whenever you feel that your mind's eye is blindfolded, breathe deeply to release all the tension that blocks your power of decision!

2. Can The AilamA® Nutrition Program provide the necessary nutrients for both sedentary and physically active people?

This eating program could become your daily diet, whether or not you are a very active person, with a deep passion for sports.

Even if you are not regularly involved in physical routines, you most likely know that physical inactivity may trigger major health inconveniencies over time.

But what if you are one of those people inconsistently engaged in physical routines, not watching their diet too closely, and still looking and feeling great?

To be sure, people that fit this profile are not fictional characters in an idealistic movie, and you may be one of them yourself.

Does this seemingly peculiar reality contradict most of the established theories on diet and nutrition? It seems so. But then again, that's real life – or what a hormonally balanced person should look like.

Being different is not a reason for grieving but for rejoicing! You don't have to hide your particularities, trying instead a largely recognized recipe for harmony. You are loved just as you are! Show your true self to the world so you won't have to fight your way to happiness.

3. Can The AilamA® Nutrition Program be a weight-loss program?

The answer is *yes*, whether you work out regularly or not. If your goal is to get slimmer, then you will definitely lose weight.

The basic principle of losing weight is to burn more calories than you eat.

A healthy nutrition program should be an eating plan that you can follow for the rest of your life, not just a 28-day-or-so diet that makes you (wish to) return to your old eating habits after its completion.

You certainly know that, whenever you deprive yourself of certain food groups, you put extra pressure on your mind, so you'll have to be very careful how you mentally frame dietary change.

The AilamA® Nutrition Program contains ingredients that can regulate your metabolic rate, thus helping you get back in shape, if needed, according to these three body types: endomorph, mesomorph, and ectomorph.

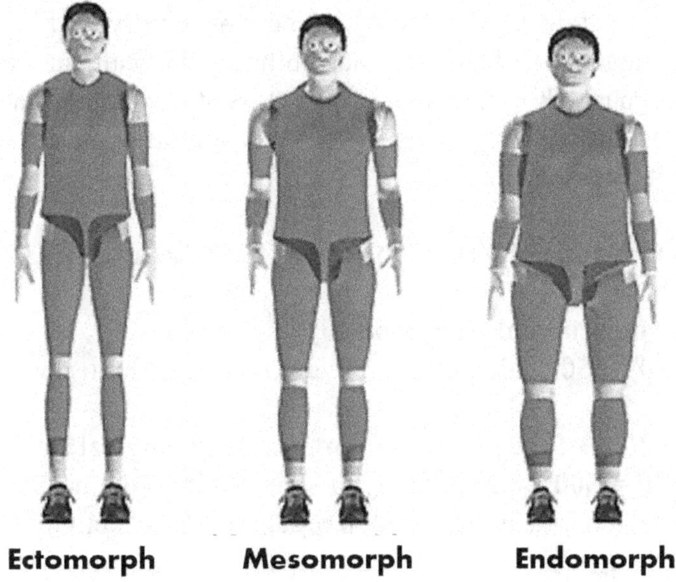

Following are important nutritional data connected to the general principles of losing weight:

a. Your resting metabolic rate (RMR) represents the amount of calories your body burns, while at rest, for vital activities such as heart beating, temperature regulation, or normal breathing.

There are people genetically predisposed to have a fast or a slow RMR.

You can increase your RMR with the right eating habits and physical exercises.

A person who works out on a regular basis to build lean muscle mass will have a fast RMR. Consequently, you should concentrate on fat loss, not on muscle loss, as the latter leads to a slow RMR.

In other words, if you lose muscle mass, your vital organs will function on low energy levels, in which case you are prone to gain fat at least twice as fast as you normally do. That's why people who have been dieting for a certain amount of time can't control their weight when they return to their old eating habits: Their metabolism runs amok because of the sudden changes in their body weight, food intake, or food selection.

b. If you want to know statistically **how much fat your body has**, do this simple calculation:

$$\text{Your Body mass}/(\text{Your height})^2 = \text{the amount of fat on your body}$$

Worrying values are to be considered starting with 25.
If you are not an athlete, you should also be worried if your figures come below 20, as they indicate that you are too thin, thus putting your health at risk.
But then again, your body is much more than a series of cold-hearted statistical assumptions!
If you are content with your current looks, make no unnecessary changes! Just be confident in your individuality and live your life accordingly.

c. Below is **the formula of losing 1 pound of body fat a week** (3500 calories):

- **Multiply your current weight by 10**
e.g. 150 lbs x 10 = **1500 calories/day**, if you don't want to lose weight

- **Calculate 20% of the above amount**, for daily physical activities
e.g. 20% x 1500 = **300 calories/day** you should add to the normal 1500 calories/day, if you are engaged in regular physical activity

- **Add 300 to 1500 calories/day**, if you are engaged in regular physical activity
e.g. 1500 + 300 = **1800 calories/day** you should eat to maintain your 150 lb weight, if you are a very active person

- **Subtract 500 from** either **1500** (if you are a sedentary person) **or 1800** (if you are a physically active person) to see **the amount of calories you should eat** if you want to **lose weight**.
e.g. 1500 - 500 = **1000 calories/day**
       1800 - 500 = **1300 calories/day**

Although calculations show that a sedentary person's body needs only 1000 calories a day to function properly while losing weight, you shouldn't go below 1200 calories/day.

The main purpose is to lose weight and be healthy! You can be thin yet you can have digestive disorders or other body dysfunctions. Don't sacrifice your health for the sake of aesthetics! Even if you may be slightly or significantly dysfunctional at the moment, your body type can still tell you all you need to know about your actual lifelong dietary needs. You can achieve and maintain a healthy body weight on an eating program that can help you shed fat, give you an energy boost, and increase your endurance capacity.

Critical calorie deprivation may lead to permanent sensation of hunger, tiredness, or dizziness.

All healthy recipes should focus on maintaining the acid-alkaline balance in the body, also called the pH of the human body.

4. Should I eat less food a day if I want to lose weight?

Restricting your food intake will never be a long-term solution, and temporary nutrient deprivation won't solve your weight problems either.

Conversely, you should concentrate on eating healthier foods, which can provide your body with the daily amount of necessary nutrients, rather than fasting! (Although *intermittent fasting* seems to be the solution to all problems for some people!)

It has been scientifically proven that you can't be healthy in the absence of these six classes of food substances: carbohydrates, fats and oils, proteins, minerals, vitamins, and water. Thus, leaving out one class while exaggerating the intake of another, even for a short time, can be both risky and dangerous.

Here is the amount of calories of the following nutrients in a gram:

- 1g carbohydrates = 4 calories
- 1 g fat = 9 calories
- 1 g proteins = 4 calories

Healthy nutrition means a balanced intake of protein, carbohydrates, and fats.

Research in this field has shown that **the best percentages of** the **macronutrients** are as follows:

- **Protein**: 30% of your daily amount of necessary calories
- **Carbohydrates**: 60% of your daily amount of necessary calories
- **Fats**: 10% of your daily amount of necessary calories

5. What if I get bored with The AilamA® Nutrition Program?

Always remember that you eat in order to be healthy.

And also keep in mind that only a happy mind can run and maintain a functional body.

When you experience moments of culinary boredom, you could indulge yourself by trying something new, whatever that may be, in small or moderate portions. In time, your body will find harmony and balance, craving only healthy food.

6. How do I know how many carbs to eat daily?

It's actually quite easy to answer this question. The rule of thumb is that the higher your fitness level is, the larger your daily intake of carbohydrates should become.

You can safely consume the same amounts of proteins and fats for longer periods of time, but your daily carbohydrate intake requirement pretty much depends on your energy level fluctuations.

Thus, if you feel dizzy or experience loss of concentration, it may be a sign that you should eat more carbohydrates.

If you have digestive problems, such as feeling bloated after meals or experiencing heartburn, your body may be quite toxic due to high acid levels and pH imbalance of the blood. In this case, you should decrease the amount of carbohydrates per day while making sure you eat more alkaline foods while eliminating the foods that may trigger over-acidification.

When your body is toxic, your liver is dysfunctional. As a result, you will feel sluggish and tired. Moreover, you can experience skin problems such as dry skin on elbows; brown spots on the body and face; acne, or itchy rash. Your tongue may be coated with a white film, especially in the morning. White spots or ridges may also appear on your fingernails, in case of severe malabsorption.

If you pay close attention to your body, it will always tell you what to eat in order to be happy, healthy, and harmonious.

7. How much water should I drink daily?

This is another question for your body to answer promptly.

Nothing could be more individual than the amount of water you need to drink on a daily basis in order to maintain perfect health.

Here are some important rules regarding your body water balance:

a. **Do not resort to any extreme measures**, like overdressing for physical exercise or overexposing yourself to high temperatures, in order to help your body eliminate excess water. The only result you will actually get is severe dehydration, which is so detrimental to your health.

b. If **the color of your urine** is dark yellow, you may not be drinking enough water, although there may be other, health-related, causes for dark urine color. If your body is dysfunctional, you need to see a qualified health care professional for a more accurate diagnosis.

If your urine is light yellow or straw yellow, then you are drinking enough water.

Clear urine color usually means that you are overhydrated. This is nearly as dangerous as dehydration, since drinking too much water can flush not only toxins out of your vital organs, but also important minerals and vitamins from your body, thus triggering further imbalances. Consequently, water is stored outside the cells (extracellular water), leading to edema (unpleasant puffiness), swelling, and inflammation.

If you press your index finger against any of your fleshy parts and have the skin slightly discolored where you are pressing down, you most certainly have water retention.

c. Plain water is the best choice to keep your body **properly hydrated**.

Also, sliced oranges sprinkled with natural salt help maintain the body's electrolyte balance. Caffeine and alcohol, on the other hand, work against proper hydration.

d. Prolonged **dehydration** causes the body to retain large amounts of water as a measure of survival.

In the morning, you can drink a glass of plain warm water on an empty stomach.

Don't drink water during meals, since it dilutes the digestive juices in your stomach. You can drink it about 30 to 45 minutes either before or after your meals.

Teas or other healthy beverages are not supposed to replace the amount of water you need to drink a day.

8. Why do I lose weight very quickly only in the first weeks?

You should definitely take into account the answer to this question if you want to stay constantly motivated throughout an eating program that regulates your weight.

At the beginning of your meal plan, nutrient-dense foods will act directly on your body, balancing your metabolism and normalizing the functions of your vital organs. As a result, you will eliminate all the water surplus from the body tissues. Your scales may not record significant weight changes during this time, but you will certainly look slimmer and fitter.

On the other hand, fat is much heavier than water, so it requires more time to be burned. That's why it becomes more and more difficult to shed a few pounds, after the first weeks. You can't lose more than 2 pounds of fat per week, but you can eliminate up to 5 pounds of water per day, if needed.

Eating less fat doesn't necessarily lead to shedding body fat. However, eating bad carbohydrates will definitely lead to storage of fat due to the hormonal imbalances all processed foods can trigger in time.

9. How does the principle of burning more calories than you eat apply to the people who are genetically predisposed to being either thin or obese?

Calorie calculation is not the only way of dealing with weight loss, or weight gain, when necessary.

The only truth that should really matter is this: A healthy body will always have an ideal weight. The word *diet* should refer to a healthy way of living, which is actually the root meaning of this versatile word.

You are healthy only when your body, mind, and soul are in harmony. All three facets of your being are interconnected!

Your metabolism and endocrine system are genetically coded responses to your inner and outer environment. For instance, if you have been exposed to stressful experiences lately, your hormonal system may be seriously affected, in which case no eating regimen can work properly, regardless of how well mapped out it is to meet your dietary needs.

Try to stay mentally and spiritually healthy in order to attain physical health and keep weight under control.

The AilamA® Nutrition Program could become your long-term meal plan, if your being resonates with its underlying principles.

10. Should I eat snacks during the day?

It depends on the types of the snacks!

However, only your individuality can give a proper answer to this question.

If you don't have a sweet tooth, you probably seldom crave sweets and chocolate.

If you feel like nibbling every two hours, you may have a fast metabolic rate, so your body may need more fuel to stay healthy.

There may be times when you snack thrice a day and there may be other times when you don't snack at all. Either way is healthy, if that's what your body is telling you to do.

If you exercise regularly, you will need to increase the intake of good carbohydrates and proteins, for energy and growth.

You can tell the difference between compulsive eating disorder and healthy frequent eating by the way you look and feel.

Always listen to your whole being and you will know when and what to snack on!

No matter how frequently you eat between meals, try to keep your liver as happy as you can! This is the first step in regaining your perfect health (in case you have lost it somewhere along the way) and maintaining it for life.

Yet, also keep in mind that no matter how well we may be eating, our liver can't be completely toxin-free simply because of the air we breathe.

The ideal scenario would be to live in totally unpolluted environments and eat only organic food prepared in the healthiest way possible. But even then we may have trouble with our own minds, which could pollute our wholeness with harmful thoughts.

So we should all be realistic and do the best we can every day to be as healthy, happy, and fulfilled as we can.

11. Should I be taking supplements?

An eating program based on healthy, nutrient-dense food should provide you with all the nutrients you need in order to achieve and maintain perfect health.

Before taking any dietary supplements, you should know exactly which organic or inorganic chemical compounds, such as carbohydrates, proteins, fats, vitamins, or minerals, you may need to supplement.

Running certain blood tests may not always be effective enough to determine correct daily supplementation with micronutrients.

Have you been taking vitamins and minerals lately? Are you still feeling weak during the day and sleepless during the night? Now you know why.

Take dietary supplements only if you are absolutely sure you need them!

A good nutrition program can help your body flush out toxins and give you energy for the whole day.

12. Can The AilamA® Nutrition Program help me get rid of cellulite?

Well, that's a tough one!

This overused term designates a dysfunctional condition of the human body, which may be the result of physical, mental, and spiritual imbalances together.

Usually, adrenal exhaustion leads to estrogen dominance along with gallbladder, liver, pancreas, kidney, or/and thyroid dysfunctions – in short, it leads to serious hormonal imbalances, which, in turn, may lead to a dimpled and/or saggy appearance of the skin.

Statistics show that there are people who have had cellulite since their early childhood.

Therefore, this skin condition may be regarded more as a genetic predisposition to hormonal imbalances rather than as simple fat storage.

A healthy diet coupled with regular exercise can definitely help you reduce cellulite in a natural way, but to completely get rid of this unpleasant condition is just a matter of individuality combined with positive thinking.

13. Should I use only organic ingredients when following The AilamA® Nutrition Program?

The terms *natural* and *organic* are sometimes used interchangeably, although they have different meanings, both of which related to the more general phrase *healthy foods*.

Natural foods contain only ingredients produced by nature or derived from animal products. However, in most countries, the term *natural* is usually replaced with the term *organic* or *bio* when the plants have been grown or the animals have been raised in a totally chemical-free environment.

If your favorite supermarket or health store sells organic foods as well as natural foods, you should definitely go for organic!

Organic foods are the healthiest, usually grown on farms that use only organic fertilizers. Moreover, organic foods are not refined after harvest. Practically, anything can be organic, from fruit and vegetables to different types of meat.

If you really want to change your life for the better, stay away from all processed foods, which have little nutritional benefits and contain different toxic chemicals to enhance their taste or extend their shelf life.

If you can't afford to buy organic foods all the time, as they are usually more expensive than the other foods, at least make sure you wash your fruit and vegetables thoroughly before using them, preferably with sodium bicarbonate.

As to regular meat, just remove its skin and fatty parts, then keep it in hot water for 5-7 minutes before using it in your dishes.

14. Can I use The AilamA® Nutrition Program for longer than four weeks, if I feel it's beneficial to me?

This eating program is ideal for fit people who want to maintain their healthy body composition.

Because of the small quantities needed at each meal, it's also perfect for the whole family so that you won't have to cook different dishes for others, but share the same meal with them, meat or no meat.

If your digestion is visibly improved and your body properly energized after having tried The AilamA® Nutrition Program, you might consider incorporating The AilamA® Recipes into your own eating regimen or making your own combinations based on The AilamA® Nutrition Program.

15. How can I tailor The AilamA® Nutrition Program to my own needs, if I want to stick with it?

You must have figured out by now what junk food is. So, if you feel like it, you can give up some of your old eating habits and create new ones, inspired by The AilamA® Nutrition Program.

If you want to lose weight, reduce your serving sizes by ¼ from Day 1 to Day 5, then increase your serving sizes by ¼ during the weekend, that is on Day 6 and Day 7.

If you want to gain weight, increase your serving sizes by ¼ from Day 1 to Day 5, then reduce your serving sizes by ¼ throughout the weekend, that is on Day 6 and Day 7.

If you feel dizzy or hungry during the program, increase your food intake as you consider it appropriate, regardless of your final goals.

Conversely, if you feel stuffed after meals, reduce your serving sizes according to your real dietary needs.

16. Can The AilamA® Nutrition Program help me overcome emotional eating?

Emotional eating is usually associated with the craving for certain foods triggered by stress, stress relief, or negative feelings such as sadness or boredom. It is usually followed by feelings of guilt or dissatisfaction, so a strong willpower may be needed to overcome this type of hunger.

Physical hunger, on the other hand, is the biological way of nourishing the body whenever there is a need for macronutrients and micronutrients. The body usually gives certain signals when blood sugar decreases below normal levels or when the stomach is empty. But in order to recognize them, we should always understand our own bodies and believe that eating for replenishing nutrients is the only healthy way of eating.

Emotional eating constitutes both an individual and a collective response to internal and external triggers.

If eating when not hungry is the all-encompassing definition of emotional eating, then the quantity of the food items consumed on such occasions should come second in importance.

Repeated snacking throughout the day, relaxing in front of the television with a huge bowl of popcorn on our lap after a stressful day at work, bingeing on fruit while reading a gripping book – these could all be forms of emotional eating if real hunger is not present.

Thus, both healthy and unhealthy food could be considered comfort food when we are stressed or when we try to regulate cortisol levels in a mechanical way.

Willpower is scientifically defined as the conscious capacity to avoid daily temptations and gratifying indulgences while following long-term goals. Since it assists in dealing with detrimental impulses, feelings, and thoughts while creating a balance between the cognitive and emotional systems, willpower plays a major role in overcoming emotional eating.

Even though bounded rationality is the most realistic type of reasoning involved in the decision-making process, willpower and self-control can always help us recognize and satisfy our physical hunger.

However, studies show that willpower is a limited inner resource, which suffers depletion throughout the day. Like any physical muscle, it grows tired when overused, while withstanding repeated temptations, which reduces its capacity to resist yet more temptations in the near future.

Low willpower can thus create special cerebral patterns in people exposed to all kinds of temptations.

On the other hand, regularly exercising willpower may lead to a much stronger self-control in the long term.

All research on willpower and self-control indicates, indirectly or directly, how important a healthy lifestyle actually is to prevent energy depletion and decision fatigue.

But, at the same time, it takes a lot of resolve to improve the quality of life, with all the temptations out there, chipping away at the self-control reserves of even the most determined people.

The brain functions on glucose, which may be easily depleted when exerting sustained self-control. Maintaining the right levels of glucose in the blood throughout the day, thus avoiding insulin spikes or insulin resistance, may help overcome emotional eating.

Willpower can also be restored by respecting the circadian rhythm and the necessary hours of restful sleep, as well as eating healthily only when hungry.

Other important ways to reboot a depleted willpower consist of consciously employing a positive mindset and belief system, adopting motivational and incentivizing behavioral patterns, and focusing on one resolution at a time, instead of many at the same time, whenever possible.

Although the decision-making process puts a toll on the daily stores of willpower, we can all find creative ways to avoid culinary temptations rather than resisting them in order to preserve our energy and avoid choosing foods by impulse.

On the other hand, fully embracing our emotional eating could help us redress, in time, this uncontrolled pattern of behavior.

So, as contradictory as it may sound, The AilamA® Nutrition Program can help you overcome emotional eating through sincere acceptance and healthy bingeing.

When there are no culinary interdictions, you will stop being reactive to forbidden food at a subconscious level. In time, your body will relearn to differentiate between physical and emotional hunger, just because you will feel no mental barriers whatsoever when it comes to the right time to eat.

Emotional eating can be both mindful and mindless, and it can also be intuitive!

The AilamA® Cookbook and Nutrition Program can help you to stop blaming yourself for eating uncontrollably and to start accepting the wonderful truth that you are both an emotional and an intuitive being.

It's like fighting fire with fire!

17. What else should I know before embarking on The AilamA® Nutrition Program?

The AilamA® Nutrition Program has been mapped out to fuel your (preferably active) body and regulate its functions. It will also orient your body toward healthy eating habits without strict measurements and calorie counts and, most importantly, without denying your emotional response to food.

You can always change the proposed amounts of ingredients to fit your own preferences and dietary needs.

If you choose to cook large quantities yet you have nobody to share your meals with, you can repeat the same day of The AilamA® Nutrition Program until you finish eating all the cooked food proposed for that day (wok, sushi, soup, bread, cake, etc.).

If you have a poor digestion, you can take half a teaspoonful of dietary fiber, i.e. psyllium seed husks, with a glass of plain water, in the morning. You can then have your breakfast, after half an hour or so.

If you are a vegetarian, just leave out the meat, plus all the other ingredients that don't go well with your life options. In this way, you will have a nutrition program tailored to meet your own dietary and emotional needs, to which you are free to add any foods or ingredients of your choice.

Always listen to your heart, the true captain of your trinity: body, mind, and soul!

ALWAYS REMEMBER

TO STAY GREAT !

Aimee T. L. Kathartt,
holistic psychologist, behavioral economist,
internationally certified sports nutritionist,
master trainer of yoga, Pilates, step-aerobics, and fitness

9 781652 190455